TITLE PAGE

Amazing
Joseph N. Geraci

DEDICATION

THIS BOOK IS DEDICATED TO ALL THE BRAVE WOMEN WHO HAVE HAD OR WILL HAVE BREAST CANCER.

TO ALL THE ORGAN DONORS AND THEIR FAMILIES BY THEIR SACRIFICE AND SELFLESSNESS THOUSANDS OF LIVES HAVE BEEN SAVED.

GOD BLESS ALL OF YOU.

INTRODUCTION

Introduction

If this were a fairy tale, the appropriate beginning would be "Once upon a time." Unfortunately it is not. *Amazing* is the true account of my wife Terry's fight with breast cancer followed by heart failure, which lead to the insertion of a left ventricular assist device (LVAD) and finally a heart transplant. This is the story of one incredible little lady. She's my little Timex "takes a licking and keeps on ticking.*[1]" She is the wind beneath our wings. Five times with the Lord's assistance she cheated death. I share with you not only the medical aspect but our daily life. I deal with our ups and downs, the anger, the joy and disappointments. *Amazing* is based on my journals, email updates and notes I jotted down while we lived this Odyssey.

I'm sure you can imagine the difficulty for each of us: Terry, the patient; myself as the well spouse and caregiver; and our daughters, Kelly and Nikki; Nikki's husband, Sean Parker, and our granddaughter, Olivia. Our world changed forever the day we learned of Terry's diagnosis

2

of breast cancer. Little did we know what the future held and where it would take us. At each point in this journey we were fortunate for professionals, family, friends and complete strangers who came into our lives at just the right moment. I firmly believe this was orchestrated by the good Lord.

In *Amazing*, you'll share the last holiday we celebrated in peace before the diagnosis, to the ensuing and weary roadmap of marital strife, nasty arguments and reconciliations that the diagnosis sent us on. Cancer puts a tremendous strain on a family, and unless you've been there, you have no comprehension as to how much. At the time we were married for almost 40 years and came within moments of splitting. *Amazing* is how we came together, resolved our differences, rekindled our marriage and now, we are closer than ever before.

After she survived cancer, you will see how the chemotherapy and radiation destroyed Terry's heart, causing the congestive heart failure that eventually led to a heart transplant. *Amazing* is the story of how one remarkable little lady faced five life-threatening events and survived to live another day.

ACKNOWLEDGEMENTS

Acknowledgements

If not for all the prayers of hundreds if not thousands of people and especially the grace of God, Terry would not be with us today.

There are a number of people I wish to thank starting with Terry's primary physician, Dr. Grace Stonerock, for being so firm and blunt with her and my primary physician, Dr. J. Patrick Tokarz for all his help and advice throughout this entire journey. I'd like to thank Inova Fair Oaks Hospital's Interventional Radiology Unit and the ICU Unit nurses; Prince William Hospital ICU Unit nurses and staff; and Dr. Eric Thorn, Virginia Cardiovascular Associates. I am grateful to the Inova Heart and Vascular Institute at Inova Fairfax Hospital with its entire staff, from the receptionist and housekeeping, to all of its wonderful doctors, and the absolutely fantastic ICU nurses; a special thank you to Cardiologist Drs. Shashank Desai and Christopher May; thoracic surgeons Drs. Nelson A. Burton, Eric L. Sarin and Anthony Rongione; the VAD Nurse Coordinators

Tonya Elliott and Lori Edwards; and heart transplant Nurse Coordinator Mary Beth Maydosz.

Above all I thank the organ donor and her family. Without their ultimate sacrifice and gift of life this book would not have a happy ending. They will forever be in my prayers.

Joe Geraci

PREFACE

Preface: The Couple on the Wedding Cake

To set the stage for the amazing story I'm about to tell you, I need to let you know a little bit regarding my wife Terry and I.

I was born Joseph Nicholas Geraci in 1947 in Buffalo, New York. I started fixing things when I was only 10 years old. A friend of my dad's, a French Canadian carpenter who lived in Fort Erie, used to come over to do punch out work for builders. He needed a helper, so I'd be his gofer. By the time I graduated Bennett High School, I hired on as an apprentice to a screw machine operator.

My life changed that summer.

I already knew Teresa Maria Nasca. Her brother Cosmo was my best friend, and I hung out at their house a lot. Cos and I would get off work, go for a swim in their pool and of course, Terry's mom had me stay for dinner. They were a Sicilian family, like mine. Cos and I understood when summer was over and we both turned 19, we would be drafted.

I asked him, "Hey, Cos, would you be upset if I took

your sister out?"

"No, not really. Go ahead."

"Well, you know, this is only a summer thing," I said.

"Nah, that's all right."

That entire summer of 1966, Terry and I were inseparable. Even when her sorority rented a cottage for a week at the lake, I slept on the beach and hung around the porch, just to be near her.

In September, we parted. I left for basic training and later that fall, I went to Air Force Technical School in Amarillo, Texas but in my heart I knew she was the one.

Dad arranged the engagement ring for me. I flew home on a three-day pass, arriving in time for Christmas Eve dinner at her family's house. We sat silently on the couch while my father, following Italian tradition formally asked her father, on my behalf, for her hand in marriage. I presented the ring to Terry and large celebration followed everybody was happy. I still tease her, how she got a diamond that broke the bank, not to mention the cost to fly home to propose to her, and all I received from her was the *Snoopy vs. the Red Baron* record by The Royal Guardsmen.

We were married at Holy Spirit Catholic Church in Buffalo NY in May 1968 with a large reception in Niagara Falls, NY. We moved to Roanoke Rapids, North Carolina, were I was stationed barely surviving on my $237.38 Air Force pay and both of us working two jobs when our daughter Kelly was born in April 1969. Nikki arrived in 1973.

I finished college at the University of Maryland while working full time as an Air Force recruiter and using my annual leave to do remodeling jobs. I could make more money in two weeks of finishing off a basement or renovating a kitchen, than I would for the whole year. The extra income helped us purchase a townhouse in Alexandria.

In 1977, I resigned from the service. Terry's dad, Jack Nasca, wanted me to come to work for him at a car dealership. I told him no. He got mad and wouldn't even talk to me. I started G&B Home Improvement with my good friend Don, a naval officer. When he transferred out, the company became Joseph's Home Repair and Improvement. I renovated historic houses in Old Town Alexandria and won two National Contractor of the Year awards. The company grew to 49 employees and 17 trucks, and there wasn't a Kay's Jewelers, J.B. Robinson or Black, Starr & Frost build out or remodel in the metro DC area we were not involved in. Even my father-in-law had to concede, "It looks like things have turned out okay for you."

Work wasn't always smooth sailing. I took on a partner who didn't work out. Dissolving the relationship took a toll on me, and in 1996, I got up one night and started coughing up and passing blood. Terry drove me to the emergency room and the doctors determined I had too much stress.

I closed the business and went on sabbatical. Terry, of course, wondered if I was ever going to go back to work. I did a few remodeling jobs for former customers, and it got to be fun again. In 1998, after reading *The Starr Report* about President Clinton and the Lewinsky affair, I joked with Terry, "Hey, what do you think if I start a company called My Rent-a-Husband? We had a good laugh, but after I did some test marketing through my BNI [Business

Networking International] group, I lined up 18 projects. So I started the business and I've been making a living off My Rent-a-Husband for 14 years now. My tag line, "I finish what your husband starts, doesn't start, and in most cases, screws up!" came from my clients.

In 2000 we moved to Manassas, Virginia. I'm probably the only person who buys a brand new house and the day after I move in, tear out the kitchen to remodel it.

Kelly married, divorced and settled in Manassas with our only granddaughter, Olivia. Nikki married Sean Parker and lives in Fairview, Pennsylvania, where she is an athletic trainer for the county school system and they both run Pentagon Paintball. They have four dogs, which I call my granddogs.

Terry and I enjoy doing many activities with Olivia. One time, I chaperoned her elementary school field trip to Washington, DC. We visited the Lincoln Memorial and the National Museum of American History. Upon our return home, Terry asked, "Well, Olivia, how was it?"

"Oh, Granny," Olivia said, "Poppa embarrassed himself."

"Why? What do you mean?"

"When we got to the Viet Nam Memorial," she whispered, "he was crying."

Terry hugged her. "Olivia," she said, "One day you will understand."

CHAPTER 1

Part One: Breast Cancer

Chapter 1: Cancer Diagnosis

The year 2007 started like any other. We had our seven-year-old granddaughter Olivia for the New Year's holiday after she spent Christmas with her dad and his family. We opened presents as if it was Christmas morning and spent the day helping her play with her new toys, games and of course, the Lionel train layout that occupies half of the family room at the holidays. We shared a great day.

Valentine's Day quickly followed six weeks later; it was the last holiday my wife Terry and I shared before our world turned upside down. We exchanged cards and kissed each other goodbye as we both left for work. We went out for a nice dinner at our favorite restaurant in Old Town Manassas, City Square Café, owned by our dear friends, Susanna and Robert Barolin. We returned home, opened a bottle of wine and shared a very romantic evening.

Later in the month, Terry went to see Dr. Stonerock,

her primary physician, for her annual physical. Terry had not followed her recommendations for a mammogram and a colonoscopy after her last physical. Thank God Dr. Stonerock firmly told her, "If you don't have both tests done before your follow-up visit with me in May, you will need to find a new doctor."

Terry scheduled the tests for March. While preparation for a colonoscopy is not the most enjoyable experience in the world, the test went well and results were negative. Next came the mammogram. Terry had annual mammograms since she turned 40. In 2006, she kept postponing the test due to work, family commitments and the holidays. This time, as always, she went alone; however, this turned out not to be a normal test. After doing the screening once, the technician told her they would need to do it again, as the imaging was blurred. After the second one was finished, the technician informed her that the radiologist wanted to speak with her before she left. The radiologist explained they found a suspicious area in her left breast. He advised her to see a surgeon and gave her several names of surgeons in the area.

Terry scheduled an appointment with a surgeon whose office was near our home in Manassas, Virginia. I went with her to the appointment. The surgeon explained the mammogram showed calcifications, which show up as tiny white dots, in the left breast. To me, they looked like tiny stars on a clear winter's night. Self-examination will never reveal these; only a mammogram will. That's why it is so important to arrange yearly screenings. The surgeon told us he needed to do a biopsy to determine if the calcifications were benign or cancerous. He said if they turned out to be cancerous, the next six months would be hell. Then the sun would shine and she would have her whole life ahead of her.

We scheduled Terry's outpatient biopsy at Prince William Hospital, where we arrived at 6 a.m., completed check in and sat in the waiting room until called into pre-op. After that, I waited alone. I always calculate the worst-case scenario. That way, if things go wrong, they won't be as bad as I imagined. I always try to have a positive to build on.

After the procedure, the surgeon invited me into one of the consultation rooms and informed me the procedure went well with no hitches. I asked him how the area looked inside. After all, one does not do this procedure every day and not gain a sense of what he found. He side-stepped my question, saying, "Let's wait for the results from the lab." He had the look of someone who is not very good at bluffing in a poker game. I knew the result would be positive; however, I still held out hope. An hour later the nurse allowed me in the recovery room. Terry was awake, aware of her surroundings, nervous and curious. She asked about the biopsy results. I stayed positive to keep her spirits up. I told her all went well and we would wait for the results.

Over the next few days I began researching breast cancer on the Internet. My knowledge of the disease was limited to my Aunt Millie, who had a mastectomy when I was a kid. I visited a number of websites, including the American Cancer Society, Cancer Treatment Centers of America and Susan G. Komen for the Cure, to name a few. I discovered one in nine women will get breast cancer; that there are different types of breast cancer and some are extremely aggressive. Some show up as tumors, others as calcifications. Cancer has four stages, depending on how far it has progressed.

On Thursday I was remodeling a kitchen in a client's rental home when Terry called my cell phone. She was terribly upset and crying uncontrollably. I asked her to calm down and talk to me. I thought she lost her job or something happened to our daughters, Kelly or Nikki, or to Olivia. She told me the surgeon had called her. He informed her over the phone she had breast cancer. He was leaving on vacation the next day and did not want to leave her wondering until he returned in two weeks.

Remember those TV commercials for the Cancer Treatment Centers of America with this same scenario? I thought, "No doctor can be that cold. It's an advertising gimmick." BOY WAS I WRONG! It took a while to calm her down and reassure her everything would be okay. The cancer was discovered early, Stage I. The diagnosis was bad, but the prognosis for a complete recovery was excellent. Once off the phone, I slid down the wall onto the floor and cried for almost a half hour. It sank in for the first time that I may lose my wife, my best friend, and the love of my life. I called my brother, Augie in Buffalo. We talked for half an hour. He had worked at Buffalo General Hospital for years as director of food services and was exposed to far more information about cancer treatments from the doctors and nurses he knew. Augie reassured me the way I reassured Terry. After hanging up, I compartmentalized the news so I could finish my work. I looked for the positives to build on.

That night neither one of us had much of an appetite. I held and consoled her as we discussed our options. She was really scared, not only because of the cancer, but because in Terry's family, by heredity, death came calling at age 58. Her grandfather, his two brothers and her aunt all died of cancer at that age. If you survived your 58th year, you would live into your eighties. Terry was 58.

After he returned from vacation, the surgeon met with us and reviewed the biopsy results. Using the mammogram, he circled the area he planned to remove. It measured 1.78 centimeters. Terry asked if surgery would remove all of the cancer and what the chances of a recurrence would be. He explained surgery would remove all the cancerous tissue and a portion of adjoining healthy tissue, which was 90 percent of the total treatment. Chemotherapy would add another few percentage points, and so would the radiation. The chemo concentrates on killing any loose cancer cells floating around the body. The radiation is pinpointed over the exact area where the surgeon removed cancerous tissue. This kills any remaining cancer cells. The three treatments together – surgery, chemotherapy and radiation – would bring her up to roughly 97 or 98 percent. You are not going to reach 100 percent, he explained. The short version is, there are no guarantees or warranties.

During this consultation the doctor completely ignored me, as if I was not in the room. He acknowledged me only when I asked a question. I thought this rude and unprofessional. I was to find during the cancer ordeal that this was standard practice among Terry's doctors. Upon leaving his office, he said to me, "You have to love her and support her." I would hear this phrase again and again as we moved through the ordeal. Each time I heard it, I would reason, "What do you think I've been doing for the last 40-plus years?"

We scheduled surgery for April. To add further insult to injury, Terry had to make another major decision that would permanently affect her. My wife has always had small breasts and this had an emotional impact on her personal esteem. So in the mid-1980s she decided to have breast enhancement surgery. Now, she was told the implants would have to be removed. Our medical insurance would cover new ones only if they were implanted at the time of surgery; however, no plastic surgeon affiliated with the hospital accepted our insurance. She could postpone the surgery while seeking a surgeon and plastic surgeon affiliated with another hospital that would accept our medical insurance or proceed to have both implants removed. Meanwhile, the cancer would continue to grow.

Physically she didn't endure a double mastectomy but mentally, I know she felt as though she had. I strongly believe after all she's been through, this indignity hurt her the most. I tried to brighten up her spirits by telling her if I wanted a big-breasted woman I would have married one. Besides, anything more than a mouthful is a waste. My male logic didn't help. She only wanted to be like other women, for her clothes to fit right and to look good in a bathing suit; simple things others take for granted.

The surgery went as expected with no surprises. They did a lumpectomy, which is a nice way of saying a partial mastectomy. They also removed two lymph nodes for testing to determine if the cancer had spread. The results were negative; the cancer hadn't spread. We now had another positive to build on. Over the next six weeks, Terry healed. Like a car on the assembly line the surgeon passed her off to the next department. His job was done except for follow up visits. I think of these as warranty visits. His words to me as we left his office echoed again, "You have to love her and support her."

During her recovery from surgery, Terry decided to go back to the church. We are both Catholics but not what may be called practicing Catholics. We would go to worship services for Christmas and Easter. When I went into the Air Force in 1966 my Uncle Tony gave me three pieces of advice: First, do not volunteer; second, you do not have to be in church to pray; and third, you will never find an atheist in a foxhole. Uncle Tony's second tidbit is one I follow to this day. Even though I didn't go to church, I pray almost daily.

Terry used this time to make peace with the Lord and ask for his grace and guidance. I knew what was ahead of her between the chemo and the radiation treatments. So if seeking spiritual direction would help and give her strength, I would support her decision. Terry needed to move past the "Why me?" stage. Having cancer is like losing a loved one. You go through the same grieving process. She moved between being bitter, upset and depressed. I sincerely hoped she would find spiritual solace that would help her through this ordeal.

CHAPTER 2

Chapter 2: Chemotherapy

While she waited to begin chemotherapy, Terry joined a breast cancer patient and survivor support group sponsored by the local hospital. These education and support groups are wonderful. Cancer patients and survivors coping with this disease, come together to share their stories and experiences. They give one another encouragement, love, support, and most of all, hope. No one should ever go through this disease alone. I don't care what the challenge is in life, until you walk a mile in someone else's shoes, there is no way to truly understand what that person is experiencing.

At the same time, I was unable to find a support group for spouses and significant others. Being a caregiver is very taxing. You have to take care of yourself and your job, plus you have to care for your ill spouse and everything they did when they were well.

I called the facilitator of Terry's group and asked if she could start one for spouses at the hospital or knew of one in the area. I was sure spouses like me would welcome the opportunity. She blew off my request, citing time, space and money issues. So I attempted to start one myself as a Yahoo! Group and spent some money to advertise it on the Web. I did this for about six months, but it never got off the ground. I just wanted to meet, even for a beer or to watch a ballgame and do something to get our minds off of what we were going through.

Eventually I found a local support group for caregivers and went to one of their meetings. They all were very cordial and nice. As the new guy on the block I got to go first and share my story. They listened very attentively and offered suggestions to assist me.

After I finished, they started sharing their situations. I felt like a weenie whiner. One woman was caring for a quadriplegic husband with only the help of teenage daughter. Another was a gentleman who celebrated a great day if when he got home from work he didn't have to change his wife's dirty diapers. At the end of the meeting the chapter president asked how I liked the meeting. I told her the meeting was very enlightening, but I wouldn't be coming back. She asked why. I told her, "I have a light at the end of the tunnel. I'm no way near the predicament you all are experiencing and frankly, I'm embarrassed for even being here and taking up your time." She did her best to reassure me and sincerely hoped I would return. In fact, I still receive emails inviting me to their monthly luncheons. But I never went back.

While talking with friends and neighbors they would say things like, "You know, Angelo's wife had it, talk to him," or "Talk to Smitty, his wife went through it." So, on my own, I did piece together a dozen or so guys whose wives had either survived the disease or were currently going through treatment. Talking with them, I learned a lot; like, what should we really expect with chemo? What would be the challenges both of us would face?

The most valuable information these well spouses provided was what to expect day to day. For example, I learned no matter what I do, or don't do, it will be wrong. If I place a dirty dish in the back of the dishwasher rack, she will tell me it belongs in the front. The next time, if I place the dirty dish in the front, she will tell me it belongs in the back. If I leave it in the sink, I'm a lazy bastard. It got so that whenever I would talk with any of these guys we finished each other's sentences. They knew what I was going say and *vice versa*. I also came to realize each of us dealt with the situation differently. Some were very macho; others hated talking about it. Some drowned themselves in work, while still others pampered their wives beyond belief. This one item would be the primary cause of our marital tensions, which led to our problems as a couple.

In May 2007 we met with the oncologist. To me, she was one of the coldest people I ever met. Then, as my wife was going through chemo, I figured out she had to be this cold to continue to do her job. I believe I would become that way, too, if I had to face death every day. If you allow yourself to become emotionally attached, you would be a basket case in no time. As with the surgeon, I was totally ignored throughout the visit. All of the conversation was directed to Terry. Again, I was only acknowledged when I asked a question. I felt as if I was an annoyance to these doctors.

The oncologist reviewed everything with Terry. She explained the significance of the mass at 1.78 centimeters. The doctor put it this way, if the mass is less than one centimeter, she would not have to undergo chemotherapy; if it was over two centimeters, she definitely would. But because the mass was in between, Terry would have to make the choice whether or not to undergo chemotherapy treatment.

If the answer was yes, Terry would have to undergo four chemotherapy treatments; one every three weeks, for a total of three months. The drug they were going use was called Adriamycin [see Index]. I wish I knew then what I know now about that poison. If you are unaware of what chemotherapy is, in layman's terms, it's the injection of a controlled poison into the patient. You kill the cancer cells by poisoning, but the dose is not enough to kill the patient.

Upon leaving the oncologist's office, she gave me that now familiar phase: "You have to love her and support her."

By the next week we had to make a decision. We discussed the options together and with our daughters Kelly and Nikki. Believe me, when you're trying to decide what to do, you go back and forth weighing all the pros and cons. I think the final factor that convinced my wife to have the chemotherapy was when she heard about a neighbor. Our neighbor was diagnosed with breast cancer in one breast and chose not to undergo chemo. A year later, she was diagnosed with cancer in the other breast and still, she refused again to undergo chemo. Later, she was diagnosed with stomach cancer, and that's when she decided to undergo both chemo and radiation. Today, she is a cancer survivor and is doing very well, but her story convinced Terry to go ahead and undergo chemotherapy. Terry wanted the added few percentage points of protection of not having a stray cancer cell floating around her body, looking for a new home. You do what you think is best for you, and hope it doesn't turn around and bite you.

The day came for her first treatment. I took Terry to the clinic and went back to the treatment area with her. Suzy, the nurse, requested I have a seat in a small waiting area while she prepared her. Once she was settled in, and the treatment was started, I would be able to go back and sit with her while the drug was administered.

After the treatment was started, Suzy came to me and said, "Mr. Geraci, your wife does not want you to see her like this. Will you please leave and pick her up in an hour or so?"

I followed her request and left. For her future appointments, I would do the same: drop her off and go have coffee and come back in an hour, or wait in the outer office waiting room until the treatment was over. Complying with her wishes would come back to haunt me later. Why? Because one of the side effects of the treatments is what is known as chemo brain. This is where the patient will not remember what they say or do. Their short term memory is affected by the drug, the body's reaction to the drug, or the trauma. She didn't remember saying this, so as a result, she felt I was unsympathetic and uncaring. This was another underlying cause of numerous arguments and marital strife.

By Father's Day 2007 Terry's hair was falling out at a fairly fast rate, so she decided to have it all cut off. She went shopping for a wig at a wig salon in Fairfax that the oncologist's office suggested. The insurance company would cover the cost as long as it was called a prosthetic and not a wig. I bet the terminology doesn't make sense to

you, either. Being that she is so tiny, none of the
"prosthetics" fit properly and it was making her very
upset. She purchased one from a salesperson, but even
though it was a size small, when she got home, the crown
or head cap was still too large for her head. It kept sliding
all over. So she went back to the store to return it. On this
visit, she spoke to the manager, who suggested she try a
child's wig. This solved the problem and now the
"prosthetic" fit her head perfectly. All this aggravation was
for nothing, however, because she would never wear it.
She put the wig in a drawer and that's where it stayed.

After each chemotherapy treatment, Terry would be
okay that day and the following day. The third day was a
different story. She would be totally wiped out and literally
would sleep for 23 hours straight. This is why her
remaining appointments were scheduled for Thursdays.
That way, the worst side effects would be over the
weekend and usually by Monday or Tuesday at the latest
she would be able to go back to work at SRA
International in Fairfax, Virginia, a contractor in national
security, civil government and health fields.

By the second treatment she was acting like a woman
with PMS on steroids and I didn't know how to deal with
her. Fortunately, I had a regular checkup with my primary
physician, Dr. Tokarz. I asked him if he had any advice on
dealing with the situation. He called a patient who he
knew was a breast cancer survivor and did volunteer work
with Y-ME of the National Capital Area, a breast cancer
support group. He asked if it would be okay to give me
her name and phone number. She replied that she would
be happy to help out. Later that day I called her and we
spoke for about 45 minutes. She gave me some useful

information and reminded me that she was a 10-year survivor and that some of the information she gave me may be outdated. She suggested I call the headquarters of Y-ME of the National Capital Area in Alexandria. The person I needed to talk with was the executive director. We played telephone tag over the next couple of days before we finally hooked up. She was wonderful. We talked for almost four hours. She took me step by step through what my wife was experiencing and what still lay ahead.

To share an example of how detailed she was, the executive director took me past the curtain and into the treatment room. I literally felt as though I was sitting in that chemo chair hooked up to the IV and feeling as though that poison was flowing through my veins. Having a complete understanding helped me immensely in dealing with the situation at hand.

She shared with me that Terry had lost all control of her life. Outsiders now had full control of her, determining who, what, where and why. The only things she still had control over were her home and me. I became her whipping boy. This is SOP or standard operating procedure for women with breast cancer, which is why I could do nothing right. Understanding this didn't make things easier. As much as I controlled myself, things got so tense around the house that the Italian in me would get the upper hand and I would start yelling. Then her Italian would kick in and we would have one heck of an argument. I also found that venting to my daughters didn't work either. They always sided with their mom and I was still wrong. As a result I would bite my tongue, leave the room or go for a drive.

Another aspect the Y-ME director and I talked about was how Terry felt abandoned. Friends whom she had been close to now avoided her, as if she had done something to offend them, or as if by coming in contact with her, they would catch the cancer. She was so hurt by this. Normally, once a month she'd go to lunch and shopping with a group of friends. Now, all of a sudden they omitted her. Repeatedly she asked me, "Why are they treating me this way?" Even her father took a very standoffish approach. Her sister said he told her he didn't know what to do. The Y-ME director explained that people react differently in these situations. Some are scared; others don't know how to act or what to say. All I can say is, at times like this, you really find out who your friends are. Also, people you barely know will step up and do things for you – people you would never expect to do so in a thousand years. For example coming home and finding dinner boxed up and waiting for you on your doorstep, or mowing your lawn so you'll have more time to care for her.

The final item we spoke of was the doctors' favorite little saying, "You have to love her and support her." This did not mean what I thought it meant. Initially, I took it to mean you literally love and support, like putting a roof over her head. What it really meant was, well, allow me to cover each one separately. Let's start with love. You have to be a real romantic. You need to see past the scars, past the bald head, and past the erratic behavior. I had to remember this was far more traumatic for her than for me. I especially had trouble with the bald head. I always thought Terry looked like her mom, but with the bald head she looked like a clone of her father. Every time I kissed her I felt as though I was kissing her father. The Y-ME director went on to say I really needed to do the little things to brighten her days. She said I would be surprised how grateful and happy Terry would be if I brought home her favorite candy bar or a can of cashews. Simply buying her a milkshake after chemo made her so happy. It would be the only thing that tasted good to her. On the support side, I needed to be Terry's rock, and be the shock absorber for all kinds of abuse and still be there for her. I had to keep it in the back of my mind that it's the cancer and the treatment doing this and not my wife.

Now, before you call me a hero or a saint, it's easier to preach than to practice this advice. Remember, I'm writing this in hindsight and I'm Monday morning quarterbacking. While you're living it, it's a different story. At times, I just couldn't hold up under the pressure. When this occurred, I tried to do one of two things. One, was to retreat to my office in the basement. Two, was to jump in the car and go for a drive. In either case, I would put on a Neil Diamond CD. Each of his tunes would remind me of a happier time. For example "Brooklyn Roads," would remind me growing up in Buffalo. The similarity between the songs lyrics and my childhood is uncanny. "Play Me" is a love song where two lovers become one and can't exist without each other. An example is the lyric that goes, "You are the song, I am the tune, play me." His music was my head adjuster. Please believe when I say you have to be a very strong, thick-skinned person.

Another side effect of treatment is chemo brain, which I mentioned earlier. The medical term is "post-chemotherapy cognitive impairment." Terry would do or say things and then not remember that she did it. Her comprehension was also affected. She became very frustrated when reading or while she was working. She would check things two and three times to be sure she understood it or did it right. The good news is, this disappears after you finish the chemo. In hindsight, I do believe a good portion of our marital strife was caused by the syndrome. Some people refer to it as chemo fog, too.

The one person who turned out to be my crutch during this period was Terry's cousin, Albert. Albert was a great sounding board for me. His first wife died from breast cancer and he was a wealth of information on how to deal with the doctors. He provided me the questions we needed to ask. Most of all, he told me, "You need to be assertive. Don't settle for what they tell you. Keep probing until you are completely satisfied." Albert learned from his ordeal that doctors, for the most part, don't give you the complete story. They don't lie to you, but they don't volunteer information either.

Albert's advice reminded of when I was an Air Force recruiter. I never lied to a recruit. I always answered all of their questions truthfully. At the same time, I never volunteered information either.

So keep asking questions, whether you think they are dumb or not. To put it another way, ask, ask, and ask, then when you think you've asked everything, come up with some more. Albert also taught me that when they give the standard, "We'll take good care of her," to respond with emphasis, "No, I expect you to take *outstanding* care for her."

The summer passed and in August 2007 Terry finished the chemo and had the final appointment with the oncologist, who wished her well and passed her down the assembly line toward the radiologist. Over September she again recouped, gradually building up her strength. Her hair started growing back and she began to feel feminine again.

Now we were faced with a new side effect, called burning mouth syndrome. The painful sensations are caused by chemotherapy (either the drug or how your body reacts to it), or when a person undergoes severe stress or a traumatic experience. Few doctors know what it is. Still fewer know how to treat it. There is no cure. Sometimes it goes away and other times it does not. No one in Terry's support group had experienced this. The oncologist said it should go away hopefully in less than a year. The best way I can describe burning mouth is to ask you to remember the last time you burned the roof of your mouth on a slice of pizza or other hot food. Now imagine your whole mouth burning like that every time you place something in your mouth, even an ice cube. Plus, everything you eat tastes like metallic garbage.

Four or five months later, while at her support group meeting, the massage therapist who was the guest speaker heard Terry talking about her burning mouth and came up to her after the program. She told Terry that she was trained in myofascial release massage, and could help her. She offered six free massages to Terry, because she wanted to demonstrate to the group that these massages help cancer patients. Terry figured why not, nothing else was helping. "What do I have to lose?" she said. So she started going to weekly massage appointments, learning the exercises and then doing them at home. These myofascial release massages did help after the six weeks. Her mouth was not only significantly better; she actually tasted food normally again.

While all this was happening life on home front was continuing to be tense and destructive. Tensions between us kept building, simmering below the surface. Remember, 2007 was the same year the housing market collapsed. My home improvement business dropped 45 percent virtually overnight. Money began to get tight, between the additional medical expenses and the drop in income. As a residential contractor, half my clients were real estate agents and brokers. I would go in and repair the houses either before they went on the market or after they were sold to new owners. Suddenly that market niche evaporated. As the drop in the housing market deepened, it also caused the collapse to the stock market. This severely reduced our 401ks and our stock portfolio. Being self employed for over 30 years, I learned a long time ago to keep a six month emergency cash reserve, but even that wasn't enough. As the depth of the housing crash and medical bills increased, our reserve dwindled. When you're self employed, you don't have a government safety net or 99 weeks of unemployment checks. We were on our own, at the time when Terry would begin the next phase of her treatment for breast cancer.

CHAPTER 3

Chapter 3: Radiation

In October 2007 Terry began radiation: 30 consecutive treatments, 30 minutes each, every day, Monday through Friday. The radiologist was no different than her two predecessors. I was treated the same way (ignored) and heard the same familiar line, "You have to love her and support her."

The radiologist's office was a few miles from her place of employment. The appointments were scheduled for 1 p.m. each day. We discussed it and agreed that she would go to these appointments by herself. My work was all over Northern Virginia and it would be extremely difficult for me to leave the job midday to meet her at the medical office, and then return to the job site. Again, this decision to act separately would cause repercussions for me later and add to our marital difficulties.

Radiation treatments are quantitative. Each builds on the previous one. As each week passed, the effect of the treatments began to take their toll on Terry. They drained her of all her energy and strength. She continued to work while having the treatments, which was necessary due to our finances, but further added to our problems. Each day she would come home exhausted and irritable. If I got home two minutes before her and she found me sitting on the couch, it was enough to get, at the bare minimum, a dirty look or grounds to start an argument.

After the 30 treatments were complete six weeks later, she was discharged from the radiologist and moved down the assembly line and out the door. A total of six months had passed since her diagnosis and it was time for the first follow-up appointment with the surgeon. He reviewed the results of her blood work, the new mammogram that was done and checked his surgical handiwork. She passed with flying colors. He wished her well and sent us on our way.

Several peculiar things happened during this entire assembly line process. First, I noticed that to each of the three different doctors and their physician's assistants, I was invisible. They all directed their conversations to Terry as if she was the only one in the room. They never even glanced at me unless I asked a question. Second, this invisibility seemed to spread everywhere. When I would run into a friend or acquaintance, they no longer asked how I was. "Hi, Joe! How's Terry?" they would ask instead. If we were out together, the same thing happened. I began to feel like a prop on the stage: dormant and waiting for that one moment in a certain scene when I would be called on to reveal my relevance.

Thanksgiving came, and while we were very grateful that the cancer was behind us, the discord between us was still simmering below the surface. It seemed our arguments were now erupting more frequently, sometimes daily. As New Year 2008 passed, our relationship deteriorated to a new low. The arguments were so intense, we were battling each other to see who could score the most hurtful verbal blow.

Finally one February morning, I was getting dressed and she was still in bed. I can't remember who or what started it, but we began to argue again. This time the argument took a different turn. It was not like any of the others. Instead of escalating, we both expressed the realization that we did not wish to end our marriage. For the first time we started talking, not yelling, at each other. We began to open up and actually communicate with each other.

She was extremely upset that "I was never there while she was undergoing chemo."

I replied, "I was told you didn't want me there." She couldn't remember saying that, to which I replied, "I'm not making it up. Look, I dropped you off, why else would I not stay?"

She then she told me about some comments I made at a Christmas party. She felt they were both hurtful and inappropriate. I told her I hadn't realized this and apologized to her.

Then she told me about the women in her support group. These women who completed their treatments were rewarded by their husbands with jewelry, cruises and other luxury gifts. All I did was to take her to dinner. She felt very hurt and unappreciated.

I said, "Terry, look, I would love to do that for you. But business sucks. I'm doing everything I can just to keep a roof over our heads. I haven't said anything to you because I didn't want you to worry."

I told her that I'd had to use our six month emergency

cash reserve in an effort to stay afloat. I was now selling off our stock portfolio and using my credit cards to pay our mortgage, utility, phone and insurance bills. I'd even started taking my Social Security early at 62, to help with our finances.

"I would love to buy you something special, but I couldn't afford to," I confessed. We both broke down cried and held each other.

That was the moment we decided to recommit to each other and work through our issues. Terry wanted to see a counselor and asked if I would do this with her. I agreed.

She found a family counselor in Manassas and we started going to see her together. I accompanied my wife for the first four sessions, and then after a month, Terry informed me that the counselor wanted to see me, alone, the following week. Within the first ten minutes I realized this woman had a feminist agenda. She did not want to hear my side of anything. Every time I brought something up, she immediately countered by saying I was wrong, it was my fault, and needed to do this or that to correct it. She said I was the one corrupting our marriage and if I was willing to mend my ways with her help, she would show me how to do it. I was so upset when I left I wanted to hit something, but I made a promise to Terry to do this.

The following week we had a joint meeting with the counselor. She immediately started asking questions about my dad and what kind of relationship I had with him. I replied we had a good relationship. Our biggest problem was due to the age difference between us. He was 44 when I was born; an old man in his 60s by the time I reached my peak teenage years. He was a good man often working three jobs to make sure we had what we needed, including a sound Catholic school education. His mom died at an early age and his biggest fear was he would die before my brothers and I grew up. He instilled in us *The Three Musketeers'* motto of "One for All and All for One." He knew if anything happened to him, we would take care of each other and be okay.

After I told her this, she immediately began to attack my dad and blame him for the bastard she thought I was. That's when I lost it and flung a throw pillow across the room. She informed me that this was her office and nobody exhibits that kind of behavior in her office.

"Fine," I said. "I'm out of here and I think you're a quack."

I left her office, never to return. Terry stayed for the remainder of the session and I waited in the car. When she got in the car, I told her that I wasn't going back. I would find someone else and work through this.

That evening I called a buddy of mine named Tony, who had moved to Las Vegas. Tony and his wife are Lutheran and very involved with their church. I met their pastor when they lived in our area and he seemed like a great guy. I gave Tony some background and asked if he thought his pastor would assist me in this ordeal. His response was, "I know he would be happy to." Tony even told me the best time – Tuesdays – to stop by his office.

I waited for Tuesday to come and drove over to his office. The pastor was welcoming and asked how things were going. I said, "Well, Pastor, that's why I'm here."

Over the next hour or so I filled him in on what had transpired over the last 11 months. He sat and listened. During this time, he only spoke a few words and took some notes. When I was finished he said to me, "Looks like there is enough blame on both sides to go around. If you both continue with the blame game, you will never accomplish anything."

The pastor told me I needed to forgive and forget and begin again fresh. He also felt one way of succeeding at this was to get closer to God. He asked if I was amenable to join his adult Bible study. He informed me to that the Bible studies were intended to lead a person to conversion in the Lutheran faith. Knowing I was Catholic, he asked if I had a problem with that.

I replied to him, "Pastor, I believe in the Holy Trinity, so if I do it as a Catholic or a Lutheran, it makes no difference to me."

The following Sunday evening I attended my first Bible study meeting. I found it to be not only interesting, but intriguing. He took passages from the Bible and gave a modern day interpretation of how they related to our everyday lives. It reminded me of algebra – the study of rules of operations and relations in math – in high school. While you are learning it, you think, "I will never use this in a thousand years." But once you are out into the real world, you're surprised how often you do use it.

Over the next four Sundays I attended each of sessions while Terry continued to see the quack counselor. One night at dinner she asked me if it would be okay if she joined me at Bible study the following Sunday. I said, "Sure, but I'm curious. Why?"

Terry told me she saw a change in me over the past few weeks and thought it would be good for her be there, too. The following Sunday we went together and everyone welcomed her into the Bible study group. Over the next six weeks we attended the meetings together and did our home study together during the week. Terry was going to Mass every week as well. On the drive home one Sunday evening Terry asked if I was set on converting to Lutheranism.

"Why?" I asked.

She replied that she did not wish to leave the Catholic Church and wondered if I would be agreeable in returning to Catholicism.

I said, "Sure, if it will help bring us back together."

The following Saturday we both went to confession together. It was the first time for me in over 40 years. That evening we attended Mass, and started going to Mass again each week.

As winter turned into spring in 2008, our marriage kept getting better and better. Our love was renewed, and we were extremely happy again. We were doing a lot of things together and I borrowed out of my 401k to help balance our finances and get us back on a somewhat even keel. Due to the economy and housing market not moving, I started a new business to help generate some much needed revenue. I have been taking photographs of trains since the early 1960s. Having accumulated over 3,500 photos, I decided to market them. We exhibited at train shows for model railroaders and arts & crafts shows both in and out of the area. Exhibiting allowed us to be together on weekends, to have fun and to meet a lot of great people – not to mention, it generated the additional revenue we sorely needed. We continued exhibiting together until August 2009.

I would like to add a few final comments on the difficulties couples face after a cancer diagnosis. According to The American Society of Clinical Oncology,

"Terminally ill cancer patients have a higher-than-average divorce rate, and it's almost always the husband leaving his sick wife." According to a study of the role that gender plays in so-called "partner abandonment," the Cancer Research Center found that "a woman is six times more likely to be separated or divorced soon after a diagnosis of cancer or multiple sclerosis than if a man in the relationship is the patient."

After talking to a lot of women cancer survivors, I often hear that "men are bums" or "he only cared about my breasts" or other similar comments. Don't get me wrong, I'm not saying all men are angels. Yes, there are narrow-minded bums who did only care about the boobs. Not to take anything away from the women who go through this battle, and Lord knows, these women go through hell, I am speaking as a spouse who experienced it. I will say this: For those husbands who stayed the distance from diagnosis through surgery, chemo, radiation and anything else that is included; remember these men suffered, too. I'm speaking as a spouse who ran this race. I was totally drained physically, mentally and emotionally. At that point some guys bail out. They are simply worn out. They have given all they can and nothing is left. Don't fault these guys or call them bastards. They were present when their spouses needed them. In remodeling we use to say "If your marriage survives a kitchen remodeling, then it will survive anything." I now say, "If your marriage survives cancer, it definitely will survive anything."

In May 2009 Terry came down with a cold that would not go away. I kept telling her to go to the doctor. She insisted it was only allergies and she didn't need to go. At the end of July we went to Michigan for a train show and while we were at the show, I noticed that things weren't right. She was tired and short of breath. Terry noticed it, too. Something was going on but it would have to wait until we got home Tuesday. Wednesday she went back to work and made an appointment to see her primary physician the following Monday.

I learned something years later. What I learned was far too late to help Terry's heart. Maybe it will save someone else's heart. I had an appointment with a thoracic surgeon I consulted on a problem I was having with my rib cage. His, and his partners' practice, is heavy into the treatment and care of breast cancer patients. While I sat in the lobby waiting to see the doctor, I picked up their brochure detailing all their methods and the different treatments they use in treating breast cancer. One item really caught my attention. It had to deal with the way they conducted the radiation treatments. For their breast cancer patients they did the radiation from the back of the patient and not from the front. This method prevents the heart from being damaged.

When I was called into the exam room, we discussed my problem and reviewed the results of the CAT scan I had taken. After we concluded my exam, I asked the surgeon if I could ask a totally unrelated question. His response was, "Sure." I asked if through-the-back radiation was a new treatment method. He replied, "No, that method has been around for at least 10 years. Why do you ask?" I told him about Terry and how the left side of her heart was damaged by the chemo and radiation.

He then shared with me that the reason they use this particular method in their practice is because his own father's heart was destroyed on the right side after receiving frontal radiation treatments. He survived the lung cancer in his right lung and then died from congestive heart failure.

So please, if you ever know or hear about someone who has to undergo radiation treatments, please pass this information on to them so they can make an informed decision along with their physician. If you do not take anything away from this book or remember anything about it, remember what you just read. It may just save a life.

CHAPTER 4

Part Two: Heart Failure

Chapter 4: Congestive Heart Failure

On Friday, just three days away from seeing her doctor, Terry went into the breakroom at work and slipped on water someone spilled and didn't mop up. She landed on her butt and wasn't hurt, just wet. That Monday, she went to work and was going to leave early for the doctor's appointment. After walking from the parking lot to the building and up to her office, she told a coworker, Phyllis, that her leg was burning. Terry asked Phyllis if she thought she should go up to the nurse's office or just wait to see the doctor. Phyllis said, "See the nurse first."

Phyllis offered to walk with her. Once in the nurse's office, the nurse told them to both to "have a seat." She needed to finish what she was doing. Phyllis was very assertive and said, "NO! You need to see her now!" Terry explained about her burning leg. The nurse could not get a pulse in her left foot and called 911. Terry was rushed to the hospital by ambulance. After she was on the way to the hospital, the nurse, who was also an employee of SRA, notified me, and I immediately left the job site and rushed to Inova Fair Oaks Hospital.

Upon arriving in the emergency room, I found her lying in one of the cubicle exam rooms and our daughter, Kelly, by her side. I asked, "What happened? What's going on?" Terry filled me in and said she was waiting for the technician to come and take her for an ultrasound on her leg. So we waited. Several hours later, she needed to use the restroom. Kelly took her by the arm and walked with her to the restroom. The restroom was not that close.

Upon returning, Terry said her leg was on fire. The emergency room nurse immediately summoned the doctor. The emergency room doctor was not a happy camper because she walked to the bathroom knowing she may have a blood clot. The emergency room staff immediately sent her over to the radiology department to have the Doppler ultrasound done. The ultrasound test checks for blood flow using sound waves. One thing I have found out about staff in ERs, recovery rooms or hospitals in general is that they go out of their way to make the patient comfortable, but family is another matter. I wish they would buy some comfortable chairs for the family members and get rid of those hard, straight back plastic and metal chairs. After sitting in them for two or three hours you begin to feel like the Tin Man from *The Wizard of Oz*. You need someone to oil your joints so you can move again.

After the test was complete, Terry was returned to the cubicle in the emergency room. Another doctor, an interventional radiologist, came in about 30 minutes later and informed us what the test showed.

A blood clot was located in the artery just below the left knee and above where the artery splits off and goes down the lower leg. Rather than remove it surgically, the ER doctor and the doctor from interventional radiology felt the best way to deal with it was to insert clot-busting drugs through the abdomen and down the artery.

Terry was immediately started on blood thinners to prevent her blood from clotting. She asked if she would be going home after the procedure. With a surprised look on his face, the ER doctor said, "No, you're going to be here awhile."

The radiology department staff scheduled Terry for the procedure, and around 10:30 p.m., and the radiology technician rolled her on a gurney to the radiology department. About 30 minutes later, the interventional radiologist came out to see me. The nursing staff had given me a bed in the recovery area to rest while they were taking care of her. The first thing I asked was, "Are you done? I don't believe I have been sleep that long."

The interventional radiologist said, "You haven't." Then he told me they were in the artery at the blockage, and the blood clot was far worse than the Doppler ultrasound revealed. The clot was approximately four inches long. She had a 99.8 percent blockage of the artery; her foot would not get enough blood if she started wiggling her toes. This why her leg burned with movement; she had virtually no blood flow in her lower leg.

I asked, "What about surgery?"

He explained that now they were in, surgery was out for the time being. He advised she would be immobilized for at least three days while the drugs worked to dissolve the clot. This was a very critical time. He continued by saying, "I have to be up front and honest with you. She might lose her toes, her foot or her leg." He explained that she would need to be closely supervised over the next three days and her leg totally immobilized.

Believe me, this is not what I wanted to hear at 11:30 p.m. at night. What could I say, except "Do the best you can and bring her back whole?" After that, I couldn't go back to sleep. I just lay there, praying the Good Lord would keep her safe. Around 1:15 a.m., he came out and said they were finished and would be moving her up to the ICU (Intensive Care Unit). An emergency room nurse gave me directions how to get there. It would be another hour or so before she would be settled in and I could see her. When I finally did get to see her, I discovered how serious the medical staff was about immobilizing her. She could not move any portion of that leg, foot or toes. Any movement might mean losing of a portion or all of her leg below the knee. I filled her in as to what happened, kissed her good night and went home.

When I showed up at the hospital on Tuesday, the ICU technician was drawing more blood for testing to help determine what caused the clot. Now, and later, I would be amazed at how much can be determined from the various blood tests they run. For now, I was told by the cardiologist that blood clots in the arteries are not a common occurrence. The majority of clots normally form in the veins. They needed to find the cause. Something was going on with heart, but what?

The electrocardiogram (ECG or EKG) revealed some irregularities so the cardiologist ordered an echocardiogram. The technician who was administering the test hooked Terry up and began the echo, but about halfway through, she suddenly left the room. The next thing I knew, Terry's ICU nurse and a cardiologist on duty were in the room overseeing the echocardiogram. Both of them remained until the test was completed. The cardiologist monitored the echo all the way through. After the test was done, he informed us of the results.

The output of her heart ejection rate was only 20 percent, meaning her body was not only oxygen deprived, but the blood was moving through the heart so slow it was clotting inside the heart. More tests would have to be run. The cardiologist ordered the necessary test required to determine what was causing her heart to underperform this way. I spent the day with Terry. She was uncomfortable and tired of being strapped in the same position, unable to move. Later in the day the test results showed some movement in the blood clot and her toes and foot were pink and healthy. This was a great sign at this point. I went home.

Upon returning to the hospital on Wednesday morning, I found my wife all bubbly and happy. I asked, "What happened?" Terry told me she had a weak pulse in her foot. This was fantastic news. It meant the blood clot was dissolving and more blood was reaching her leg and foot. Now we had to wait on the results of all the blood work and the other tests they ran. Later in the day we started getting the test results.

The news was not bright. The diagnosis was serious. Terry had congestive heart failure caused by viral cardiomyopathy. Her abdomen and chest and ankles were full of fluid. The medical staff needed to start reducing the fluid levels in her body. A kidney specialist was brought in to monitor her kidneys and their output. A regimen of diuretics was started to bring down her fluid levels. The cardiologist started medication to improve the output of her heart while the kidney specialist monitored fluid levels and the condition of her kidneys. Over the next eight days she would lose almost a gallon and a half of fluid, or roughly 12 lbs. of water weight.

Thursday brought us great news: the clot was dissolved and the artery was open. Terry now had a very strong pulse in her left foot. The cardiologist ordered the use of the medications to improve her heart's output. Basically, the hope was to mend her heart to an acceptable level. She spent a total of ten days in the hospital and at the conclusion, the heart medication was working. The final echocardiogram showed her heart ejection rate had increased to 25 percent. The cardiologist believed her heart was severely weakened as a result of the chemotherapy and radiation treatments.

At the time of her chemotherapy and radiation treatments, both her oncologist and radiologist told us these procedures had a one to two percent chance of damaging other organs. They said not to worry, it's a very small percentage.

The cold that wouldn't go away that spring was the straw that broke the camel's back and sent her heart over the edge. The fall she took at work actually was a lifesaver. The cardiologist, the interventional radiologist and the internist who were treating her all believed the impact when her butt hit the floor broke the clot free and sent it south. Normally when this type of arterial clot breaks free it goes northward. It travels up the aorta to the brain and certain death.

Over the next several months, Terry continued the new regimen of drugs and visited the cardiologist monthly. Her heart's output had improved to 40 percent by the end of October. This was good, but not great. She was still working and carrying a full schedule. Terry has always been an avid reader. She would always have a book in her hand. Now she was not only too tired to read, but when she did she had trouble comprehending what she read. By the time we finished dinner she would be totally exhausted and would go to bed. On weekends, she spent most of the time sleeping and resting. I gradually assumed more and more of the household duties. Generally speaking, Terry had always taken care of the inside of the house and me, the outside. Now I was doing it all. A friend of ours put it this way: "How do you like being a single mom?"

Up to this time I was always a very sound sleeper. I never heard our kids crying when they were babies. While I was in the Air Force I even slept through a wing of B-52s taking off and landing. Now I would wake up with the slightest change in her breathing and I would check to see if she was okay. I was her first line of defense if something happened.

Our Fall 2009 Arts and Craft Show season started. Terry no longer helped me work the shows because they were just too taxing on her. To put this in perspective for you, I was doing a local show and forgot my lunch at home. I called and ask if she would run it over. Her walk from the disabled parking place into the hall and down to my booth wiped her out. She arrived huffing and puffing, totally out breath, and it took almost a half hour for her to recover.

As Christmas 2009 approached her health continued to worsen. As each day passed she had less and less energy. She would be out of breath walking from the car into the house. Every time we mentioned this to her cardiologist, he would say, "Everything is okay, the EKG is good." This cardiology practice has the reputation of being one the best in the Washington, DC metro area. They're lucky we haven't sued them for malpractice.

By the end of February 2010, Terry no longer walked up a flight of stairs without stopping four or five times. To walk across our kitchen, she needed to stop twice to catch her breath. I remember very clearly, it was the first Friday in March 2010. Terry was scheduled for her monthly cardiologist appointment in the morning. I also scheduled an appointment for her with my pulmonary doctor, Dr. Foley, for the afternoon.

At the appointment with her cardiologist, we informed him about her shortness of breath. Actually she was huffing and puffing as he was examining her. Plus her abdomen, ankles and feet were swollen. She had an almost continuous cough; she wasn't sleeping well and she was gaining weight again.

Yet he said to us, "The EKG is good and your heart sounds good. I can hear a little fluid. You have nothing to worry about. As for the breathing, you need to see a pulmonary specialist."

That's when I said, "We're doing that in the afternoon."

Later that afternoon we saw Dr. Foley my Pulmonary Doctor. She examined Terry, checked her blood oxygen level and administered a breathing test. Afterwards Dr. Foley met us in her office to share the results. Terry failed both tests big time. Something was definitely going on and she wanted to schedule other tests for the following week. One of the possibilities could be lung cancer; she mentioned this because of Terry's history of breast cancer. A cancer cell might have survived and taken root in her lungs. Also, a number of her family members had died of various cancers.

Dr. Foley said, "Let's wait until all the tests are completed. Then we will have the answers." She gave Terry several inhalers to use to help her breath better.

As our luck would have it, we didn't make it to any of the tests the following week. Monday evening after Terry returned from work, she changed her clothes and came downstairs for dinner. She was having a very hard time breathing. She needed to stop and catch her breath after every step. When she reached the kitchen she said to me "I cannot do this anymore". I told her, "Get your coat, we're going to the emergency room."

As soon as we got to the emergency room at Prince William Hospital the ER staff immediately took her into an exam room and hooked her up to oxygen. Dr. Eric Thorn, the cardiologist on duty, was called in. Dr. Thorn was so young looking, I swore he was a high school student. As a cardiologist, he is the absolute best IN MY BOOK, a super, super doctor. He literally saved Terry's life. He examined her and looked at the results of the EKG. She was having severe congestive heart failure and was admitted again to the ICU unit.

Over the next several days a variety of tests were ordered. By Thursday, all the results were in. Dr. Thorn arrived early that morning to give us an update. What he told us was not good. Terry's liver and kidneys were shutting down. Toxins were building up in her body; she was full of fluid in her chest, abdomen and ankles. The echocardiogram showed her heart ejection rate was now between 10 and 15 percent. Putting it perspective, she was two heart beats away from a pine box.

The top priority was to get her stable. The catch-22 was that with the condition of the liver and kidneys, the removal of fluid throughout her body and around her heart was not going to be easy. Dr. Thorn ordered a kidney and liver specialist to be brought in.

Terry was in no way getting anywhere near the amount of oxygenated blood she required for her organs to work properly. At the same time, because her heart was so weak, the medical staff was worried about any additional strain being put on the heart by her liver and kidneys. The staff would monitor her liver and kidneys very closely to be sure she would not have complete renal failure. Whatever needed to be done had to be accomplished very carefully and very slowly. Her heart would not handle it any other way.

Dr. Thorn presented me with a loose-leaf binder on congestive heart failure. The information included sheets listing all of the symptoms, causes, treatments and long-term prognosis. The major symptoms are shortness of breath, coughing, abdominal swelling, fatigue, weight gain, trouble sleeping and swollen ankles. Sound familiar? This is exactly what we told her former so-called doctor of cardiology less than a week earlier and he told us her heart was fine. How that idiot ever made it through medical school I will never know.

Under causes, I discovered another interesting tidbit. The #1 cause of congestive heart failure is chemotherapy; the #3 cause is radiation. Earlier, both the oncologist and radiologist had told us there was only a one or two percent chance of damaging other organs. I immediately wondered, "How can that translate into the #1 and #3 causes of congestive heart failure?" I can't tell you how many websites I researched, looking for studies on the relation between the two. I was never able to find any. I have concluded these doctors pick the one or two percent chance of chemotherapy or radiation damaging other organs out of their hat. Nowhere could I find a study that looked at X number of cancer survivors who underwent chemo one year, three years, five or ten years later to follow up and see how many actually developed organ damage. If they have, they are hiding it pretty well. I did find a paper published and copyrighted by the American Association of Cancer Research in 1977. It documented an experiment completed on rats for Andriamycin-induced Cardiotoxicity (Cardiomyopathy and Congestive Heart Failure) in Rats.[2] The researchers found that the majority of rats treated developed Cardiomyopathy 3 to 23 weeks after the last injection.

As we progressed through this journey, we learned that heart failure is measured in four stages, from Stage 1, the mildest, to Stage 4, the most critical and life threatening. Both Dr. Thorn and later, Dr. Shashank Desai, described it this way. As a patient moves from one stage to the next, the length and frequency of days spent in the hospital for treatment steadily increases while the health, heart function and quality of life progressively worsens. At this point, Terry was in Stage 2, borderline Stage 3. When a patient reaches Stage 4, death is not far behind unless they receive a transplant.

My family and I will always be extremely grateful to Dr. Eric Thorn and all the nurses and technicians of the ICU Unit at Prince William Hospital. Their efforts brought Terry home to us. When she left the hospital she was stable and her organs were still oxygen-deprived, but functioning properly.

At her April 2010 appointment, Dr. Thorn suggested Terry have an ICD implanted. An ICD is an implantable cardioverter-defibrillator. The main killer of congestive heart failure patients is heart arrhythmia, which causes the heart to beat uncontrollably or the heart just stops. The ICD was intended to prevent this from happening.

Dr. Thorn went on to tell us the latest test showed the medications were not working any longer. Her heart ejection rate was hovering at 20 percent. It had not changed since she left the hospital. What he said next startled both of us: "I've used all the tools in my tool box. You need to think about a transplant."

We both simultaneously said, "What?"

Dr. Thorn emphasized again that he had done all he could. Now was the time to seek those who could still help her survive.

The surgery to implant the ICD was done as an outpatient at Inova Heart and Vascular Institute at Inova Fairfax Hospital in early May 2010. Dr. Sanasari, one of Dr. Thorn's associates, did the procedure.

After the surgery, we now faced having to make a much bigger decision about the heart transplant. For the next month Terry and I talked about it, discussing the options. However, when we looked at the bottom line, the only choice was either, "Do I want to live?" or "Do I want to die?"

At her May appointment we discussed the transplant at length with Dr. Thorn. In the end, we agreed that the referral to Inova Heart and Vascular Institute at Inova Fairfax Hospital in Fairfax, Virginia, was definitely the next step. One thing really worried me about the journey we were about to start on, and that was Terry's blood type. Terry is AB positive, which is very rare. If she needed a transplant I wondered if she would ever get one as a result of her blood type.

Up to this time, Terry was still attending the breast cancer support group meetings. When she started to discuss what she was currently experiencing as a result of her cancer treatments, the group turned against her. These were negative effects that the members did not want to hear her talk about or even know about. She understood by their comments that they only wanted her to share positive thoughts. In fact, several of the group members told her that what she was telling them was bringing the group down. Terry explained that she just wanted to make the group aware of what might happen as a result of these treatments. She wanted to increase their awareness and provide them with information so maybe they would not suffer what she had endured. The group members wanted no part of it, and as a whole, made her feel very unwelcome. Terry stopped attending the meetings, and to this date she has not returned. I sometimes wonder how many of these group members could have benefited from what she had to share with them.

Terry's first appointment at the heart center was scheduled for early June 2010. Shortly after arriving there, we were called in and met a lovely young nurse by the name of Carliegh. She took Terry's medical history and reviewed all of the medical records forwarded by Dr. Thorn's office. We then met Dr. Christopher May, one of two transplant doctors at Inova Heart and Vascular Institute at Inova Fairfax Hospital. Dr. May examined Terry and asked if we had any questions. I'm sure you can bet what my first question was. His answer was that being an AB blood type, she was a universal recipient, meaning that she would be able to receive any blood type organ: A, B, AB or O.

After hearing that, I was so relieved. Once all our questions were answered, Dr. May informed us the first thing that needed to be done was to have a heart catheterization. He went on to tell us that once you have congestive heart failure, it doesn't go away. There is no cure. The heart muscle has been damaged, and over a period of time it only gets worse. The heart catheterization procedure, which would be done as an outpatient, would determine the exact condition of her heart. This was scheduled for June 15. Being new to this, we figured they would perform the test, then we go home. Wrong!

Once the test was done and we were informed of the results, our lives changed again as we knew it. It felt as though we were on a leisurely Sunday drive in the country and suddenly found ourselves in the middle of the Daytona 500. The test revealed the pressures inside the left side of her heart were very low. Plus her heart output (ejection) was only 1.2 liters of blood per minute. The normal heart's output is 5 to 5.5 liters of blood per minute. Basically, if she sat in a chair and didn't move – only blinked – she would have enough blood to keep all her organs happy. Any movement or motion and she would suffer from oxygen deprivation.

Terry was admitted to the hospital and started on a drug called Milrinone. The drug is administered through an intravenous PICC (peripherally inserted central catheter) line inserted directly into the heart. Milrinone makes the heart work and squeeze harder, thus pushing out more blood. It is a short-term fix. Eventually one of two things happen: the heart either stops totally or the heart becomes immune to the drug. It's like taking a whip to a horse. The horse will react in one of two ways: "the hell with you!" and not go any faster or at some point it will just stop.

Over the next several days I learned how to change the

IV bag and prime and run the pump. Terry would have to live with the pump 24/7. She would carry a small bag that contained the IV bag and pump. It was like carrying a second purse over her shoulder. She could not be discharged from the hospital until we received the necessary supplies from the company our insurance company used. I was contacted by the "in home" company and they shipped the equipment and the medication overnight. Plus they assigned a nurse who would be available to us 24/7. Once I received the supplies, I brought them to the hospital so Terry could be discharged. While still going through the discharge process we were contacted by Judy. She would be Terry's home nurse. Terry made an appointment for Judy to meet with us at the house for later in the afternoon. Judy was wonderful.

CHAPTER 5

Chapter 5:   The Left Ventricular Assist Device (LVAD)

While Terry was in the hospital the doctors started talking about an LVAD. I know you're thinking, "a what?" An LVAD is a Left Ventricular Assist Device. Basically, think of it as a mechanical heart, but not quite. You probably saw news reports about former Vice President Dick Cheney, who was an LVAD recipient in July 2010 before his heart transplant in March 2012. Both surgeries were performed at Inova Heart and Vascular Institute at Fairfax Hospital. Or you may have read about Ally Smith Babineaux, the young woman *People* magazine called the "Bionic Bride" after the Texas Medical Center installed an LVAD in the 22-year-old in 2010. Babineaux, who was also diagnosed with viral cardiomyopathy, underwent a heart transplant in 2011.

Basically, I think of the LVAD as a fifth or sixth generation Jarvik-7, but not quite. The Jarvik-7 was the artificial heart retired dentist Barney Clark received in 1982 at the University of Utah. He survived 112 days after surgery.

Actually the LVAD is a battery/electrically operated, computer run, centrifugal pump. A 5/8" hole is cut into the bottom of the left ventricle of the heart. A fitting is sutured to the heart and then a hose attached to the pump is connected. The other end of the pump also has a hose attached. This hose runs up to the aorta where a second hole is made and second fitting is sutured to the artery. Then a second hose from the pump is attached. The pump also has a driveline. The driveline is run through the abdominal cavity and exits through the skin on the right side. The drive line is connected to a computer connected to two external batteries or a base unit powered by electricity. The doctors set the pump at 8900 revolutions per minute (RPM) to start. Afterwards, the medical staff monitors both the patient and the LVAD. The RPM can then be regulated up or down depending on the condition of the heart and the height and weight of the person. Another interesting fact about LVAD patients is, you no longer have a pulse or blood pressure. If you listen to the chest with a stethoscope, all you hear is the whirling sound of the pump.

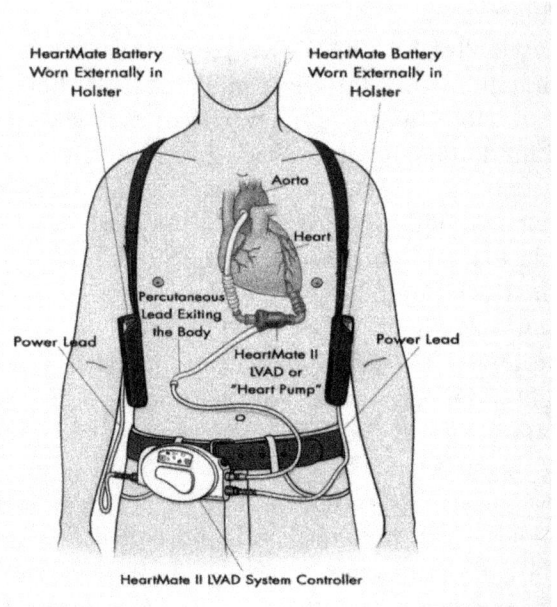

Illustration of the HeartMate II® Left Ventricular Assist Device (LVAD), courtesy of Thoratec Corporation.

The VAD Coordinator Lori Edwards came to visit us in the hospital and starting talking to us about the LVAD. We learned that there are two models by two different medical device manufacturing companies. One is the HeartMate II® by Thoratec Corporation (used by Cheney and Babineaux) and the second is HeartWare® by HeartWare International, Inc.

At the time of Terry's diagnosis, the HeartMate II®, had approval of the Federal Drug Administration (FDA). HeartWare® was considered experimental because the medical device company was in the testing for FDA approval. HeartWare® is a miniaturized unit, about the size of a cell phone. The batteries and computer are also smaller and lighter in weight. This was the unit they wanted to place in Terry because of her small size (at 5', 125 lbs., Terry is very petite). Because this unit was still experimental, however, the transplant doctors did not know if our insurance would cover it. If not, they would reapply for the HeartMate II®.

So Terry and I had to learn about each model unit. We were given two 1-1/2 inch loose leaf binders, one on each of the LVADs, spelling out everything. I took one home to read while Terry read the other in the hospital. The next day we switched binders. We needed to learn how each of the two devices worked, the pros and cons, all of the different health warnings and the potential dangers of having a LVAD. Just because either pump would furnish the needed blood to your body, they did not come without risk. Besides the risk you encounter with any major surgery, now we are dealing with open heart surgery on a damaged heart. Plus there would be a chance of a stroke that could be major. The blood could clot and build up on the fins of the pump, causing it to stop.

After reading both binders, I have to tell you honestly, I don't know if I would have decided to proceed if it was me. To me, it was like reading the paper that comes with a prescription drug. After learning all the warnings and side effects, you wonder: Do I really need to take this drug? Will it do more harm than good?

While Terry was in the hospital we had consultations with a social worker, a financial advisor and a dietitian. Each had to chime in. The social worker needed to sign off on Terry's attitude and support system. Was her attitude positive? Did she want to have the procedure done? The support system is critical. After the patient has the surgery and the pump is installed, the patient would need to be cared for 24/7 during the first weeks at home, with someone changing the dressing on the wound daily. After that, it would be at least three months before her driving privileges are reinstated. The financial advisor discussed our insurance coverage and issues. The dietitian reviewed nutrition. She instructed us on how to live on a low-salt, low-fat diet and showed us ways to spice up and improve the taste of food without adding salt. She also discussed what foods should be avoided to maintain a low-fat diet, especially all processed foods. We were to avoid fried foods; but if we did fry something, we needed to use olive or canola oil only.

We joined the hospital's heart and lung transplant/ VAD heart support and education group. Both of us wanted more knowledge about VADs (there are right ventricular assist devices or RVADs as well) and what other patients felt about them. The people in this support group were the most upbeat, positive people you ever would want to meet. They not only drew in strength from each other, they all offered it back as well. We wanted to learn day-to-day information about living with the VAD, what problems they experienced, and how they resolved those problems. The hospital staff and the binders give you all the technical and medical information, but they can't give you the inside, personal accounts of what life is like living with the VAD. The group members provided us a wealth of information. They were always there to support each other and provide each other ways to make living with the VAD easier. For example, one woman shared a resource: She found a lady in Bay City, Michigan, Cindy Bosco, who designed the Bosco LVAD Vest so her husband, Phil, could carry the equipment more easily and comfortably. The LVAD's exterior equipment weighs almost eight pounds. Plus when you leave home, you need to carry two spare batteries and a spare computer with you, adding another eight pounds. Bosco was marketing the vest on her website, www.boscolvadvest.com. Even former Vice President Dick Cheney had used one of her vests.

Through the binder and the support group we learned that during the day the LVAD runs on two batteries that last approximately 12 hours on a charge. The unit comes with a battery charger and eight batteries. At night you're connected to a power base and monitor. This base unit has a 20-foot tethered line to allow you to move around the room. The monitor shows the RPM, the output of blood in liters and the power level. In the group, they talked about changing your home to make things easier for the LVAD patient. For example, just getting up at night to use the bathroom can be a challenge. If the tether line is too short to reach the bathroom, the patient has to come off the tether and go on batteries. Any time a part of the system is disconnected, an alarm will sound, waking up anyone in hearing distance. When returning to bed, the patient needs to switch back to the base unit. In case you are wondering, you can't sleep with the unit on batteries. The patient has to be connected to the base unit. The base unit has an emergency backup battery built-in. In case of a power outage in the middle of the night, the patient will be alerted and have sufficient time to change over to batteries.

Terry was discharged from the hospital and for the next seven weeks she was on the Milrinone. Each week Nurse Judy, Terry's home health nurse as she referred to herself, would come to the house to take Terry's vital signs and draw blood. She would also check the PICC line for infection and change her dressing. Judy was always available anytime day or night. If I had trouble or a problem I just called her. Of course these calls never came between normal business hours. One night I called her at 11:30 p.m., because I was having trouble changing the IV and I didn't want to break the plastic connections. She walked me through it and told me what tools I could use to loosen the connection without damaging anything. Another time she delivered replacement pumps to us in the middle of the night because the primary and backup pump alarms kept going off. She was not only a super nurse, but an absolutely fantastic individual who became a good friend.

The purpose of the Milrinone treatment was to get Terry as healthy as possible for the next step on this journey, the LVAD surgery. She had been so oxygen deprived for so long it weakened her organs. At this point Terry could no longer work and went out on short-term disability. The majority of her day was spent either in bed or on the couch sleeping. In the mornings I would make her breakfast, change the IV bag and rotate the pump. The pumps had to be rotated and batteries changed daily. After I was sure she was squared away, I would leave for work. If I was working close to home I would come home and fix lunch. Otherwise, I would make sure things were laid out for her to eat lunch. In the evening, I would fix dinner, clean the kitchen and get everything ready for her so she could go to bed. I would then wash a load of laundry, place it in the dryer, and go to bed. In the morning I would take the clothes out of the dryer, hang or fold them, and put them away. I then put another load in the washer and fixed breakfast. Once a week, I would grab the grocery list off the refrigerator and head to the grocery store. Ironically, Terry never used to let me near the grocery store. She would always say I either would buy too much or buy a bunch of stuff we didn't need. Now I can honestly say I'm a Certified Professional Shopper. I check labels, ingredients and prices. I even clip and bring my own coupons.

The fatigue and lack of comprehension Terry experienced while reading worsened. She stopped reading altogether. In fact, the hospital staff tests patients to gauge how well their brains are functioning. Terry was given a sheet of paper with the letters A to J and numbers 1 to 10 on it. The letters and numbers were randomly spread across the page. She was instructed to draw lines, like connecting the dots, from the letter A to the number 1, and from the number 1 to the letter B, and so on. She was timed, and the time it takes to finish was recorded as a baseline for future tests. Another test they performed was a six-minute walk. They measured the distance she could walk in six minutes to establish a baseline. After the pump is installed, she would be tested again after six weeks to measure improvement. An interesting tidbit I learned from Dr. Desai, the other transplant doctor at the hospital, was that the temples of the forehead of people who suffer from oxygen deprivation will become concave. Terry's temples were terribly concaved; I never noticed it before.

From then on whenever I speak to someone, I automatically look at their temples.

During this seven-week period all the rounds of doctor and clinic appointments kept us busy. Every two weeks she was examined at the clinic and blood was drawn to check a whole series of things. I am amazed how much can be determined from analyzing several vials of blood. In addition, once she was going to get an LVAD and being considered for a transplant, we needed to have everyone verify her health including her primary doctor, dentist, oncologist, surgeon, hospital psychiatrist and social worker, plus the transplant team all had to sign off. Anyone being considered for transplant has to be tested from head to toe. If you are wondering why Terry needed all these doctors to sign off, it's because first she needed to be healthy enough to undergo open heart surgery. Second, to get a transplant, her case would go before a medical committee for approval before she could be placed on the transplant list. If she was not a good candidate or they felt she would not survive the surgery, she would not be approved for transplant.

This process proved to be very interesting when we met with her oncologist. She came into the exam room, exchanged pleasantries and sat down in the chair by the little desk area you find in these rooms. The doctor asked Terry why she was there because it wasn't time for her regular six month checkup. Terry told her she was going to have LVAD surgery and she was being screened for a heart transplant. The doctor didn't say anything. She bent her arm at the elbow and raised her hand to her forehead covering her eyes for a moment then looked at Terry. Her body language said it all. It screamed OH, MY GOD,

NOT ANOTHER ONE! I firmly believe these doctors pick the one or two percent chance of organ damage out of thin air just to make the decision for chemotherapy treatment an easier sell. Personally, in the future, I would trust an aluminum siding salesman, a used car salesman, or even a politician before an oncologist or radiologist.

Normally when Terry would have a six month follow up at the oncologist's office, she'd go in, have the blood work done, and then either the doctor or her physician assistant would tell her, "Everything's okay, see you six months." Never once had they done anything else.

Now that the oncologist had to signoff so Terry could have the LVAD and heart transplant, she ordered a PET scan (positron emission tomography). This scan specifically detects any cancer in the body. Terry and I both determined this was a "cover your ass" move on her part.

After all the medical appointments were completed, we then had an appointment with Dr. Nelson Burton, the thoracic surgeon who would perform the LVAD implant operation. Dr. Burton is the Surgical Director, Heart and Lung Transplantation, for Inova Heart and Vascular Institute at Inova Fairfax Hospital. He told Terry she was going to be the smallest person in whom he had ever surgically implanted an LVAD. He continued to tell her not to worry, that he would make it fit. My understanding is, the LVADs were designed for men. It was only recently they started implanting them in women.

We continued attending the VAD support and education group meetings. Terry would always have a new set of questions to ask the group at each meeting. After attending these support group meetings we began to look at holidays differently. I know it sounds morbid, but we learned most donor organs come as a result of automobile and motorcycle accidents. Holidays were spoken of as donor days. Motorcycles were called donorcycles. It was beginning to dawn on us that someone else's tragedy was going to be Terry's miracle. I still have trouble accepting the fact that one's life is extended only by the supreme sacrifice of another. To this day, I pray for the donor and her family.

Terry's LVAD surgery was scheduled for August 16, 2010, a month after Dick Cheney received his LVAD at Inova Heart and Vascular Institute at Fairfax Hospital. Later I learned that LVADs were only implanted at two facilities in the Washington, DC metro area: Inova Fairfax Hospital and Washington Hospital Center. The hospital submitted all of Terry's paperwork to our insurance company for approval to do the surgery. That is when all the fun started. The hospital submitted it as a *bridge to transplant*. The insurance company disapproved the procedure, but not for the reasons you may think. Inova Heart and Vascular Institute was not approved as one of their Life Centers, despite the fact that they'd just done Dick Cheney's *bridge to transplant* operation, and in the past 33 years, had done more than 30,000 heart operations.

Therefore, since it was a *bridge to transplant*, we would have to travel to one of four centers with who our insurance carrier had under contract. The closest to us was the University of Virginia Health System in Charlottesville, Virginia – 94 miles away. The other choices were in Philadelphia or Pittsburgh, Pennsylvania to the north, or Charlotte, North Carolina to the south. We could not believe that they did not have a Life Center in the Baltimore or Washington, DC metro area. After all we are not in the middle of fly-over country.

If we still wanted the surgery performed at Inova Heart and Vascular Institute, we would have to do it out of network, meaning our insurance would pay only 70 percent of the total cost; we would pay the difference out of pocket. Keep in mind, we are talking about a procedure costing about a quarter of a million dollars. If we used one of their contracted Life Centers, our insurance would cover the procedure 100 percent.

Terry was upset that this would mean we would have to start all over again at UVA's medical center. She was so happy at Fairfax. She felt very secure with the blanket of doctors, nurses and staff that surrounded her there. Terry felt as though she was in the middle of a protective bubble surrounded by all these wonderful professionals. For the next two weeks I would spend my entire day from 9 to 5 on the phone with either our case manager at the insurance company, a wonderful young registered nurse by the name of Gemma Stein; the financial people and staff at Inova Fairfax, or the human resources department of Terry's employer. Everyone was trying to work out a way so the surgery could be done at Fairfax.

Now I cannot say this with any certainty – it is only a gut feeling I have – but I firmly believe her employer exerted enough influence on the insurance company to get this done. In the end, the reason for the surgery on the paperwork was changed from *bridge to transplant* to *destination*. In other words, it was changed from "the surgical implant of a device that will keep her alive until she could receive a heart transplant" to "the surgical implant of a permanent device." Kind of like the earlier run-in with the insurance company over covering the cost of a *prosthetic* as long as it wasn't called what it really was – a *wig*. This sounds simple, but it is actually more complicated than that.

Another thing I discovered was there is health insurance and then there is transplant insurance. Look at it as a railroad track with two ribbons of steel that run parallel but never intersect. Fortunately her employer, SRA International, when negotiating the contract for health insurance, included transplant coverage. I always wondered when you hear about churches or the media helping people raise money for a transplant. I would say to myself, why do they not have insurance? They probably did; only they had health insurance coverage and not transplant insurance coverage. Another example is home insurance. We all think we're covered, as long as we have a home insurance policy. But if your house gets flooded, you are not covered unless you have flood insurance as well.

Permission was granted for the surgery using the HeartMate II®. All we had to do now was wait until August 16. The week before the surgery, we received a call from Dr. Burton's office. They requested changing the surgery until August 18. Dr. Burton was returning to Washington, DC on a late flight the evening of August 15. In the event the flight was delayed he felt it best to postpone 48 hours. Hey, when you have the best, waiting another 48 hours for him is okay. This moved the date of the surgery to August 18 – Terry's birthday. What a birthday present: A new lease on life, and an opportunity to have, once again, a somewhat normal life.

After the surgery, Dr. Burton commented that it was a challenge to get the pump in place. He ended up shifting her stomach a little to make room for it.

Both VAD coordinators, Lori Edwards and Tonya Elliott, prepared our daughter Kelly and me on what to expect post-surgery. Tonya is one of my favorites at Inova Fairfax. We both grew up in Buffalo, we both are diehard Bills fans and we both have a warped sense of humor. Tonya and Lori did everything they could so we would not be scared when we saw her after the surgery. Terry would be on a ventilator, connected to 15-plus IVs, numerous other equipment including monitors, a ventilator, drain lines and, of course, her base unit, they said. They left out one thing, however: how swollen she would be. When we walked into intensive care, we were shocked. To me, Terry looked like three-day-old road kill. Kelly and I were visibly upset upon seeing her. Terry's ICU nurse kept saying, "She's okay, she's doing fine, don't worry. This is normal." I thought to myself, "If this is normal, I'd hate to see abnormal."

The next morning I returned, and wow, what a transformation. She was off the ventilator and conscious. Much of the swelling was gone. Terry's ICU nurse didn't want her to talk for a while because her throat was irritated by the ventilator. That day and every day thereafter would be very busy initially for me and then for Terry as she improved. Now that the LVAD was in, I needed to read the manuals and become familiar with all the equipment. How do I connect and disconnect the batteries? What each of the alarms signals and lights meant? Could I silence them temporarily? Both of us had to learn how to switch out the computer unit if it failed: This is the most important and crucial thing you need to know. The computer is the brain behind the LVAD; if it crashes, so does the heart. You have to be fast, accurate, and proficient. If not, someone dies. You almost need to know how to do it blindfolded. Don't worry, I wasn't practicing with her unit. You are provided with a working unit. The pump has a looped hose filled with water, two computer units and four batteries with which to play. You have to think of this procedure as holding your breath; you can only do it for so long because you are holding the heartbeat. I didn't wish to find out the time limit on that one.

When Terry would get home, I would have to change her dressing daily so I needed to learn how to do a sterile dressing change, clean the driveline, and how to waterproof the driveline incision area so she could shower. Learning this wasn't hard, except each day I had a different nurse showing me. Each had their own technique to do things and the order of steps kept changing. Eventually I learned to do it seven different ways. One day I complained to Tonya and she showed me what she called the down and dirty method. It included all the major steps without the frills.

Once while Terry was sleeping I got bored and started looking in drawers. I found the doctor's manual that came with all the equipment; it was step-by-step instruction manual on how to do the LVAD surgery! It had everything you wanted to know about the surgery. It showed the type and number of sutures and what knots to use. Plus it showed the tool used to cut the hole into the heart and aorta and how to do it. Being a contractor I found this manual absolutely fascinating. Earlier my son-in-law, Sean, was curious as to how they primed the pump. I told him I didn't know. Now I had the manual so I called him in Pennsylvania to tell him. While I was reading the manual, Lori Edwards, the VAD coordinator came in and noticed what I was reading. She said, "You're reading the wrong book."

I replied, "I know, but it's more fun. I just hope someone wasn't reading this to the doctors in surgery." Lori thought I was serious and got all flustered.

Each day Terry kept improving by leap and bounds. The number of IVs and the amount of equipment kept leaving the room. Initially she had six drain lines in and until they were all out, she could not get out of bed. One by one they would be removed until finally the last one was out and she could start walking around with help. Both the occupational and physical therapist started working with her.

Nine days after the surgery Terry was discharged – one of the fastest LVAD patients to move through recovery and out the door. The average discharge is 14 days after surgery. That made her sort of their poster girl.

As part of the discharge process there was a kind of a "final exam." The VAD coordinators go over everything with you, including testing you on the battery and computer switch out, which we both had to pass. We also were given a loose leaf binder to take home. It contains all the emergency numbers, instructions and the daily recordkeeping logs. Terry would need to record her weight, temperature and blood pressure twice a day, plus the information displayed on the base unit monitor. The book also had a section on where to go charge the batteries and what to do in an extended power outage. We would have to bring this book with us on every clinic visit.

The hospital and the VAD coordinators developed a

community outreach program. They trained and instructed all the emergency response teams in the Washington, DC metro area on how to deal with a VAD patient in a 911 emergency. All we had to do when they arrived was to say "She has an LVAD code orange." They in turn had a book provided by the hospital that was color coded. They would simply open to the orange section and it provided them all the information they required. We were told this, but little did I know I would have to use it the very next day. The VAD coordinator even notified Northern Virginia Electric Cooperative (NOVEC), our local electric provider, to let their customer service center know that Terry was on a life support system that required constant use of electrically-powered medical equipment. This meant during a power outage we were priority one.

Once we were home and settled in I went and had her prescriptions filled. That night she took them, but the next morning she felt really sick. I called the hospital to talk to the VAD coordinator on duty. I didn't want to go running to the hospital on the first day. Tonya Elliott called me back within five minutes and I explained Terry's symptoms to her. She said, "Call 911 and have her brought to the heart center." I hung up and called 911. The ambulance with emergency medical technicians arrived within minutes. Once inside the house, I said, "She is an LVAD patient, code orange." They opened the book and knew exactly what to do. When I told them she needed to go to the Inova Heart and Vascular Institute at Fairfax Hospital, I was informed they would require permission to go outside the county.

One of the EMTs called the local hospital and at first, the emergency room doctor said, "No."

The EMT replied, "Sir you do not understand; she has a left ventricular assist device."

"A what?"

The EMT repeated it. There was a moment of silence, then the doctor replied, "No one here knows what that is. Go ahead and take her to Fairfax."

Now please, do not think anything negative about the staff being unaware of VADs. At the time, there were only 100 plus people in the entire Washington, DC metro area who had an implanted LVAD.

Upon arrival at Inova Fairfax, a hospital team was waiting. They determined she was having an allergic reaction to the new blood pressure medication. We stayed for several hours in the emergency room until they were sure she was okay. Then I took her home.

After the first couple of nights, I knew I needed a plan for the house so she could maneuver better at night. The tether line was too short to go from the bed to the toilet. The manual said, "Keep the base unit away from moisture." I decided they were not talking about steam in the bathroom. So I moved the base unit between our double sinks. We also exchanged sides of the bed. I made a combination metal and plastic hanger to hang the equipment in the shower. For showering, the batteries and computer were placed in a special waterproof shower bag. The bag looks like a brief case except one side is clear plastic. It has a strap and a handle. With these changes she could now maneuver around the bedroom and bathroom without switching to batteries.

We slowly began adapting to life with an LVAD. Each day Terry recorded her weight, temperature and the information reflected on the monitor. She ran a self-test of the controller and its alarms to be sure everything was okay.

At Terry's October clinic appointment, Tonya, one of the VAD coordinators, asked Terry if she wished to take part in a VAD study. Terry had to record all her vital information daily into a log book. If there was anything out of the ordinary we would need to call the hospital. As a study participant, she received a computer terminal, a computerized scale for weighing herself, and a computerized blood pressure monitor. Each morning as she did her logging in routine, her weight and blood pressure readings were sent wirelessly to the computer terminal, which in turn called it into a central office in Orlando, Florida. From there, the data would be monitored by a nurse named Michele England. Michele was wonderful. Any slight changes to Terry's numbers and she was on the phone to ensure there was not a problem. Over the next six months, Michele became a great long-distance friend, even though we never met her. After Michele's review of the daily information, it was transmitted to the VAD coordinators at Inova Heart and Vascular Institute.

When leaving the house, we developed a check list so as to not forget anything. Terry had to change her wardrobe. She could no longer wear dresses due to the drive line; only pants, blouses and pullovers. We always tried to be home when the batteries needed to be changed. Terry got embarrassed if the batteries needed changing and we were out. One evening, we were having dinner at Red Lobster and the battery alarms went off. Suddenly, half the people in the restaurant were staring at us. They watched as I changed her batteries. When I finished, I said, "Even the

Energizer Rabbit has to have a change of batteries sometime!" Several of those diners close to us were curious and I told them about the LVAD, what it did and how it worked. They were amazed about the technology and how far medicine had progressed. Terry, on the other hand, was embarrassed by the entire episode.

In October 2010, during a thunderstorm, a lightning bolt hit a transformer located behind a neighbor's house. Besides the power being out, the transformer was sparking and burning up on the pole. I dialed 911 for the fire department. Then I called NOVEC to report the outage. Several minutes later the fire department arrived. A Prince William County fire captain knocked on our door to see if everything was okay with Terry and to see if she had enough charged batteries. I thought this was very considerate of him and I thanked him for inquiring about her. While we were talking, a NOVEC crew showed up with everything they needed to get the power back on. The foreman also came over to inquire if Terry would be okay while the repair was going on. Within three hours we had power again. This priority treatment delighted our neighbors.

Terry continued to heal but never really regained her strength and energy. She was tired all the time. She would do a little, then nap for a while. While Terry was healing, she was pretty much homebound.

Our granddaughter, Olivia, said, "Granny, you can have Buddy stay with you for as long as you want. He'll keep you company." Olivia's dog Buddy is a Pomeranian mix that my daughter Kelly adopted from the animal shelter. He's one of the friendliest little lap dogs you ever you wanted to meet. Buddy stayed with us for three weeks.

He did wonders for Terry's psyche. After our last Golden Retriever, Brandy, died in 2000, we decided not to get another dog. Now, after spending this healing time with Buddy, Terry suggested we adopt a small dog. So the search began; in the meantime, Buddy would still come and spend the weekends with us. We couldn't get Olivia to spend every weekend though. You know how those 10-year-olds going on 19 are!

Terry continued to heal in November. She regained her driving privileges and was able to get out on her own again. Her trips were short – only around the City of Manassas. I know she enjoyed having this independence again. For me, I was relieved of at least one of my duties as constant chauffeur.

The weeks turned into months and before we knew it we were in the New Year. Terry had hoped that after six months she would be able to go back to work. This never happened. At the support group, other VAD patients would talk about how great they were feeling and many had gone back to work. Terry kept wondering, "What's wrong with me?" The doctors tried to increase the RPMs on the pump. They discovered increasing to 9200 RPMs was the max they could go on her. This was the most her heart could handle without putting her in serious harm's way. [Later, after she had the transplant surgery, I asked the heart transplant doctor, Dr. Desai, just how bad her heart had deteriorated as a result of the congestive heart failure. He replied by saying, "You're in construction, you know the bricks with holes in them. That is what the left side of your wife's heart looked like." To put it another way, her heart muscle had lost its flexibility. It was very fibrous and could no longer expand and contract.]

In February 2011, nearly six months had passed since the LVAD surgery. We had our hardwood floors resanded as a result of storm damage. We needed to stay in a hotel for six days. Besides our luggage, I needed to bring the battery charger, monitor, base unit, implantable cardioverter defibrillator (ICD) monitor, blood pressure monitor, scale and all her medication. Plus I found after getting in the room I would need to go back to the house and pick up an extension cord. Unless you travel with an electric-powered medical device, I bet you never thought about the critical need for electrical receptacles in a hotel room. They are few, just enough for a lamp and clock, and not located to accommodate a VAD. We took only one other weekend trip and I was sure to pack the extension cord.

Long-distance travel became challenging as well. No longer could we just get up and go. If we wanted to leave the area, we needed to notify the VAD coordinators, give them the dates of our travel and our itinerary. They, in turn, provided us phone numbers and locations of medical centers in the area where we were traveling in the event of an emergency. They also notified the hospitals in those cities that an LVAD patient was in their area.

At the end of February, I had a total knee replacement. My brother, Augie, came down for a few days to help out. After he went home, Terry and I were like the rubber-legged comedy ice skaters Frick and Frack; between the two of us, we couldn't make one, but we made it through.

Even with the light moments, though, as time progressed, Terry began to really hate the VAD and her depression worsened. She kept saying, "I've done everything they told me to do and I'm no better. I still can't work or do anything. This is no life." She was tired of carrying all the weight around. She just wanted to hop in the shower without a 20-minute preparation. I kept encouraging her and doing what I could to cheer her up. I found what worked best was to say to her, "Don't you want to see Olivia grow up?"

In April 2011, Terry had ordered one of the Bosco LVAD Vests in beige. In late June she received it, but it was too big. Cindy Bosco called her and said another woman had returned one in Terry's size. She had received her new heart two weeks after wearing the vest. The previous owner felt the vest was lucky and wanted Cindy to pass it on and see if the good fortune would continue. Cindy told Terry if she would like it she would ship it out to her, and she did.

In June, Terry's long-term disability would be over and she would be discharged from SRA effective July 1, 2011. At the end of June, I took Terry to SRA's corporate headquarters in Fairfax to clean out her desk. I knew this was very hard on her. More than anything, she wanted to go back to work. She loved her job, the company she worked for, and especially the people with whom she worked. How often can you say that? While she was saying goodbye, she and her coworkers were all crying. She really did not want to leave.

Now that she was officially terminated, we needed to start on COBRA. Terry had been on permanent disability from Social Security effective December 31, 2010. So she made the decision to go to the University of Virginia Health System and start over to get on the transplant list. The doctors and staff at Inova Heart and Vascular Institute at Inova Fairfax Hospital understood, and would forward all of her records to UVA. I notified our case manager, Gemma Stein, at the insurance company, of Terry's decision. Gemma provided me all the contact information at UVA. She also said she would call UVA and give them a heads up. I called UVA in Charlottesville and made an appointment for May 18, 2011. Terry was happy. She had fully come to terms with her decision.

On Friday, May 13, just five days before her appointment at UVA, we received a call from Carliegh at Inova Heart and Vascular Institute. She told us that our insurance company and Inova had negotiated a contract to be one of their Life Centers, and had signed a letter of intent. Again, I cannot say this with any certainty – it's just my gut feeling – but I believe her employer again exerted pressure on the insurance company to negotiate a contract; if not with Inova Heart and Vascular Institute, then with another heart center in the Washington, DC metro area. Carliegh wanted to schedule an appointment to update Terry's file and officially have her placed on the heart transplant list. The staff at Inova Heart and Vascular Institute scheduled the necessary tests and blood work they required. After we completed these steps, we met with Dr. Burton again. He came in to interview both of us.

Dr. Burton asked Terry a whole series of questions. One question was, "How are doing, living with the LVAD?"

She replied, "I hate it. I'm tired of carrying all this weight around. It's heavy and cumbersome."

When I heard Terry's answer, I thought, "Oh, my God, you just blew your chance to get on the list."

Dr. Burton replied, "That may be so, Terry, but it has

kept you alive to reach this point."

Later that evening, while having dinner, we received a call from Carliegh. She informed us the medical committee had met that afternoon. Terry's case was presented and she was approved for transplant. We were ecstatic and thanked God for this blessing.

However, we needed to do one more thing. While at the clinic, I was given a list of all the medications Terry would be required to take after the transplant. The list was two pages long. I needed to contact our insurance provider to see if our insurance covered them. If so, how much, and what would be our deductible? I needed the prices for both the brand name and the generic brands. These drugs aren't cheap either. A 30-day supply for just one of the drugs was over $6,000. A 30-day supply of another drug was over $2,500. If the cost of these drugs was not covered, I needed to provide a financial plan showing how we were going to cover their cost. If financially you can't purchase these drugs, you will not receive a transplant. Again, thank you SRA for providing such great coverage. We learned that we would be able to afford all of our deductibles, even on COBRA.

Once on the heart transplant list you are placed in one of four categories. The *Category 1A* patient is in the CCU (Cardiac Care Unit) and is very sick, with the highest priority of their heart failing, or the patient is someone who has complications from their LVAD. The *Category 1B* LVAD patient needs a heart, or is on IV medications, but is not in hospital and, is stable. The *Category 2* patient is at home on heart failure medication. The *Category 7* patient is inactive on the list, such as a patient who is out of the area or more than two hours from the transplant center. Terry was placed on the list as a Category 1B, and her next clinic appointment was set for June 29.

Being on the list is exciting because it provides you hope. Each day you wonder, "Is this the day we'll get the call?" Before we knew it we were in the middle of Memorial Day weekend, but we just stayed around the house. Terry didn't want to go anywhere in case the call came. She has had a cell phone for years. Most of the time, she leaves it at home. Now that she was on the list, she kept that phone charged and she even bought a special holder so she could wear it around her neck. Sunday morning, as we were getting dressed, we had the TV on in the bedroom. The 1988 movie *Beaches* was playing. This movie has always been one my favorites because of the soundtrack and because I am a fan of both Bette Midler and Barbara Hershey. In the past, when viewing the scene where the doctor tells Barbara Hershey's character she is dying of viral cardiomyopathy, we thought, "Oh, she's dying of heart disease." This time, Terry and I both looked at each other. Now, we can quote you chapter and verse on every aspect of this disease.

At the June appointment we met with Mary Beth Maydosz, the heart transplant nurse practitioner. She informed us that once a patient is on the list, each patient is afforded a one-time opportunity to be bumped up to the top of the list for a 30-day period. There were still no guarantees Terry would receive a heart during this time frame. Someone else could suddenly become critical, and she would get bumped back, or a heart might not become available during this 30-day period. There would be no do-overs or Mulligans. The way it works is, the doctors review everyone within the region who is on the list for what their current medical condition is, plus other factors unknown to us, and they determine your best opportunity to receive a heart if one becomes available. Mary Beth informed us that the doctors had determined this was Terry's time. Her 30 days would start tomorrow. WOW, was Terry excited!

On the way home I told her, "Someone up there really likes you." Ever since she started this journey with the breast cancer, people we knew and met would always say they would add her to their prayers. Over this five-year period, the number of people praying for her grew exponentially. She was on prayer lists in churches from New York to Florida; from Virginia to California and all parts in between. She is a recipient of prayers from all denominations – Catholic, Baptist, Lutheran, Methodist, Presbyterian, Evangelical, Jewish and Hindu. I even had people stopping me at the grocery store or in a restaurant. They recognized my company jacket and asked if I was Joe Geraci. When I replied, "Yes," they would tell about Terry being on the prayer list at their church. I would thank them and let them know how she was doing. Even when I went to vote, and was giving my name to the election official, the woman next to her asked, "Do you have a daughter named Kelly?" When I responded, "Yes," she said, "I'm her realtor, and my church has been praying for your wife."

As the days passed and the end of the 30 days approached, Terry was becoming very anxious and apprehensive. On the evening of Tuesday, July 26, we just finished dinner and decided to sit out on the deck. As I went out the door, I grabbed the phone. I don't why, I just did. Once out on the deck Terry opened up.

"Joe, there's only four more days and we haven't heard a word. I don't think I will ever get a heart." She started crying. "I hate this VAD! Why can't I just be like other people?"

It took me a while to get her calmed down. I told her, "Look, don't give up. We still have four more days. If it doesn't happen, you're still on the list and your time will come."

I no more than finished telling her this, when the phone rang. I looked at the caller ID and it read INOVAFAR.

I knew this was the call; I didn't want to answer the phone and steal her excitement. I kept a straight face and I said, "Here, this call is for you," and handed her the phone. It was Mary Beth Maydosz. She told Terry they may have a heart. The hospital had been alerted, but we would have to wait. Mary Beth said she would call back within 30 minutes to let us know for sure. Terry was so excited, she started crying tears of joy and we just hugged each other on the deck.

One thing that has always troubled me through this whole transplant process is someone has to die to make this gift of life possible. So as I hugged her, we thanked the Lord for this gift and asked Him to spread His grace on the donor and her family. Then we sat there, waiting for the follow up call. It was like waiting for water to boil. Thirty minutes seemed like an eternity.

Sure enough, 30 minutes later the phone rang. It was Mary Beth calling again. She asked, "Where are you located?"

I said, "Manassas."

She said, "Then we will see you in 45 minutes. When you get here, go to the Third Floor Nurse's Station and the check-in. The team will be waiting for you and take you to Room 359." I grabbed all the LVAD gear, realizing that Terry was wearing the lucky VAD vest that Cindy Bosco had sent her. I commented to Terry "This vest must truly be Lucky". We left immediately. Terry called our daughters, Kelly and Nikki, from the car to let them know the news. Once at the hospital, I would call with more details.

Exactly 45 minutes later, I was pulling into the parking garage at Inova Fairfax Hospital. We proceeded up to the third floor and stopped at the nurse's station. The nurse asked if she could help us.

Terry replied, "Yes, I'm here for my new heart."

The nurse chuckled because she said she had never heard it put that way. She said she would call our nurse and took us to Room 359. Several minutes later, Terry's nurse came in, introduced herself, gave Terry a hospital gown and started the check-in procedure. We learned that the new heart was coming from northeast Pennsylvania. This was on the border of two regions and the donor's organs would be shared between the two regions. As a result, they needed to wait until all the transplant teams from both regions were present before the organs could be procured from the donor. This meant Terry would be admitted to the hospital and go into surgery either just before the night shift would go off, or just after the day shift came on. I called our girls and gave them the update. Kelly arranged to have a friend take care of the family dog, Buddy. Olivia was visiting with her Aunt Nikki and Uncle Sean. Kelly would arrive in Fairfax around 6 a.m. Nikki lives in Pennsylvania, so I would update her throughout the day.

Terry was bubbly and raring to go. She wasn't the least bit nervous. I, on the other hand, was a different story. As surgeries go, it doesn't get any bigger than heart transplant surgery. Was this going to be a dry run and we go home? How would I keep her motivated? What if they couldn't get the new heart to start? What was actually going to happen that I was not ready or prepared for?

PHOTOS

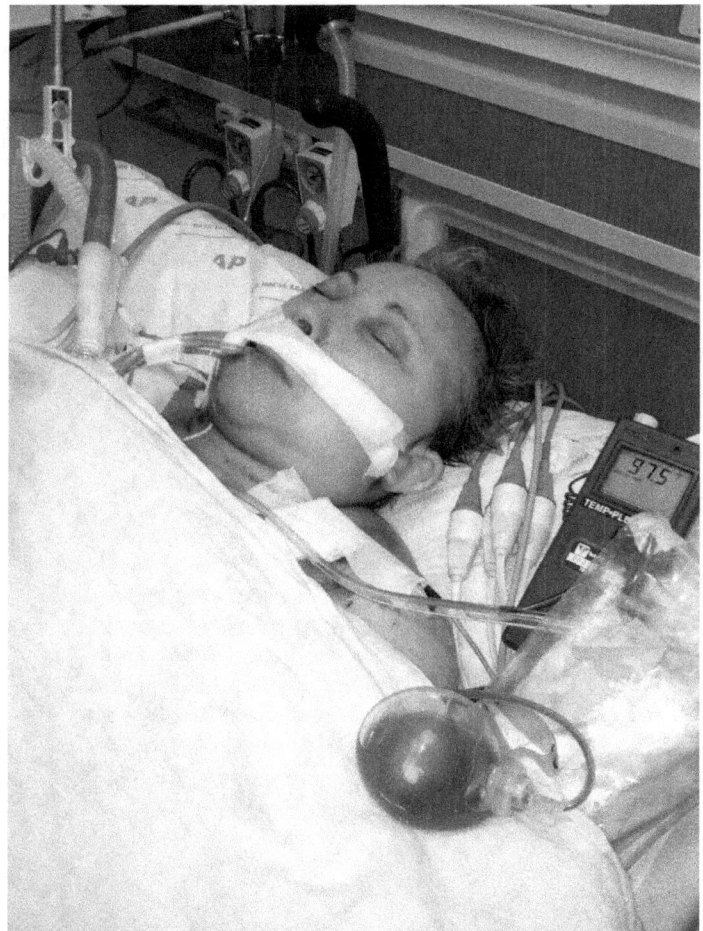

Day 2 after transplant Terry regaining her facial features, she is still severely swollen.

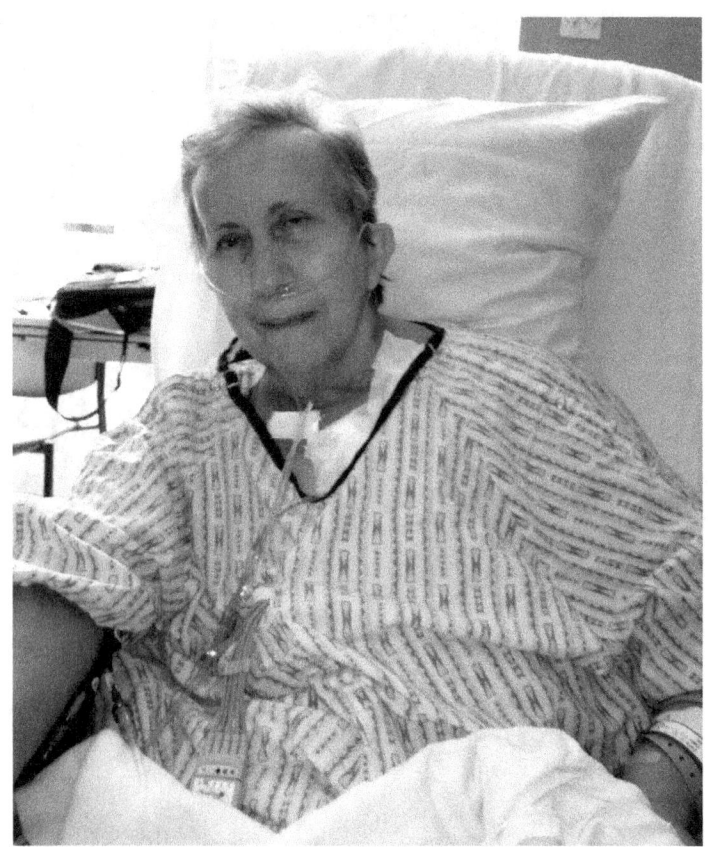

First time Terry is up and in a chair.

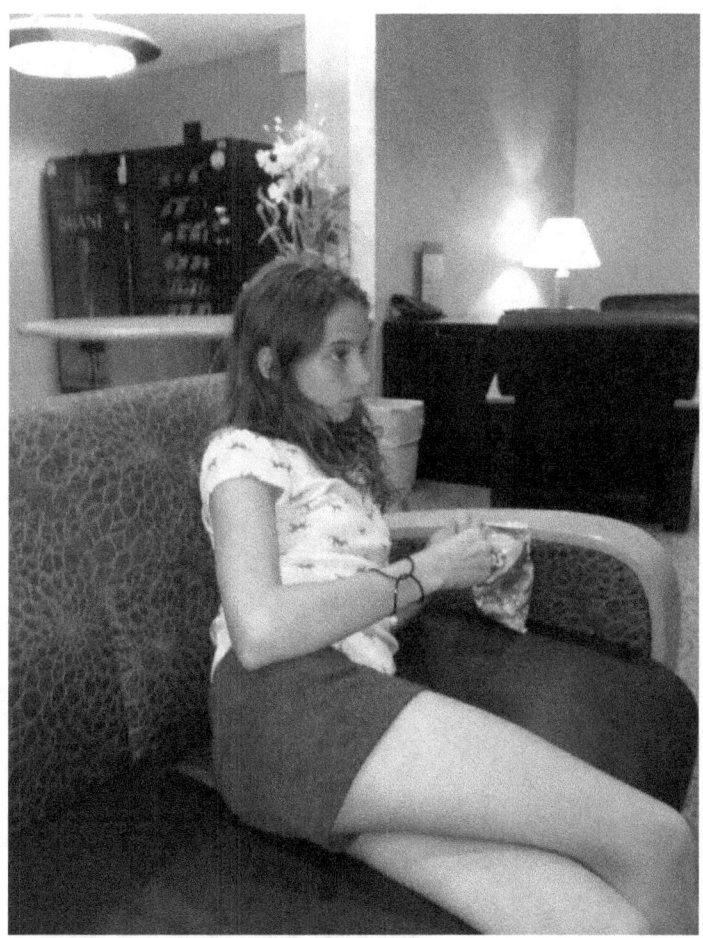

Olivia waits patiently to see her Granny.

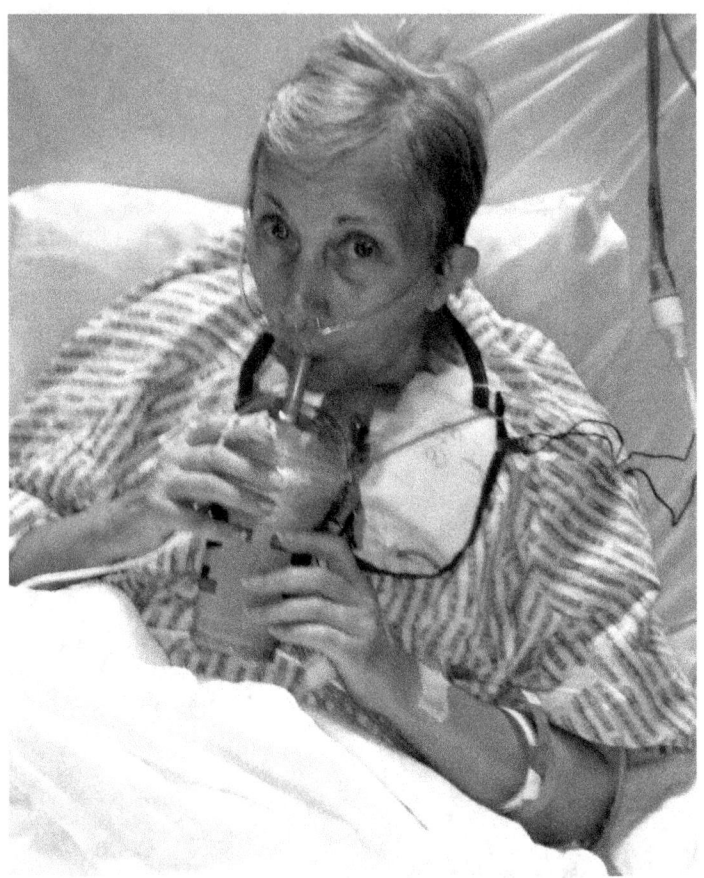

Terry Finally gets her chocolate milk shake.
* * *

Terry's ReBirthday - Hopefully the first of many with her new heart.

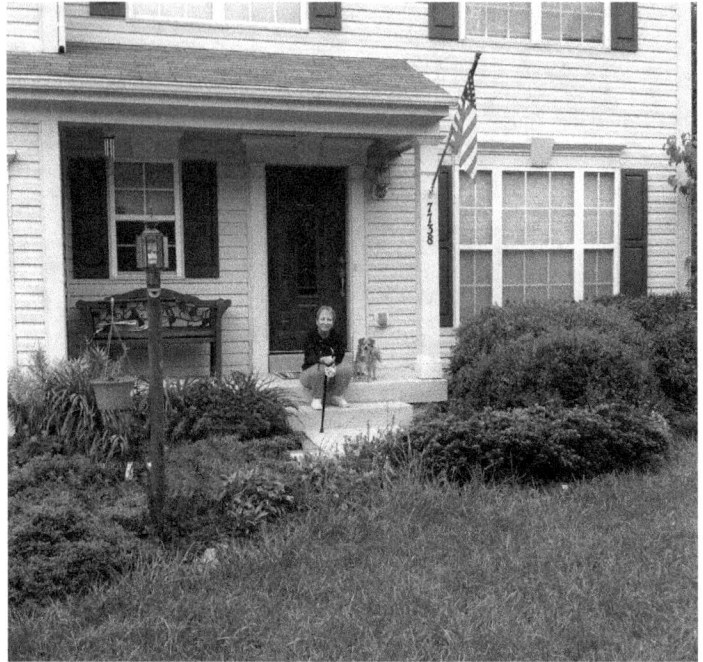

Terry and Buddy relax on the porch while Terry is confined to the house.

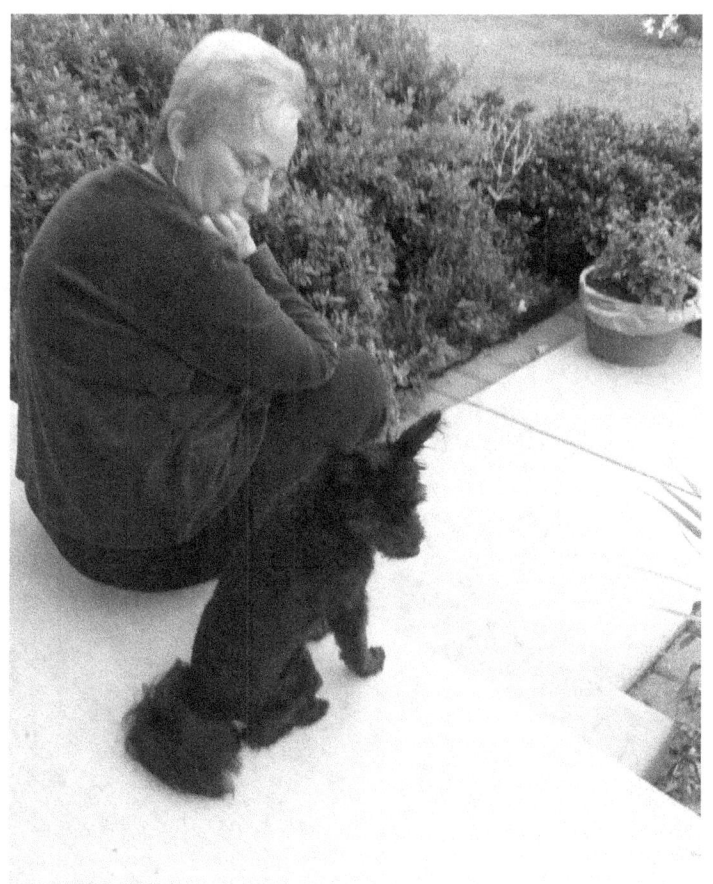

Terry and Eddie enjoy a spring afternoon after returning home.
* * *

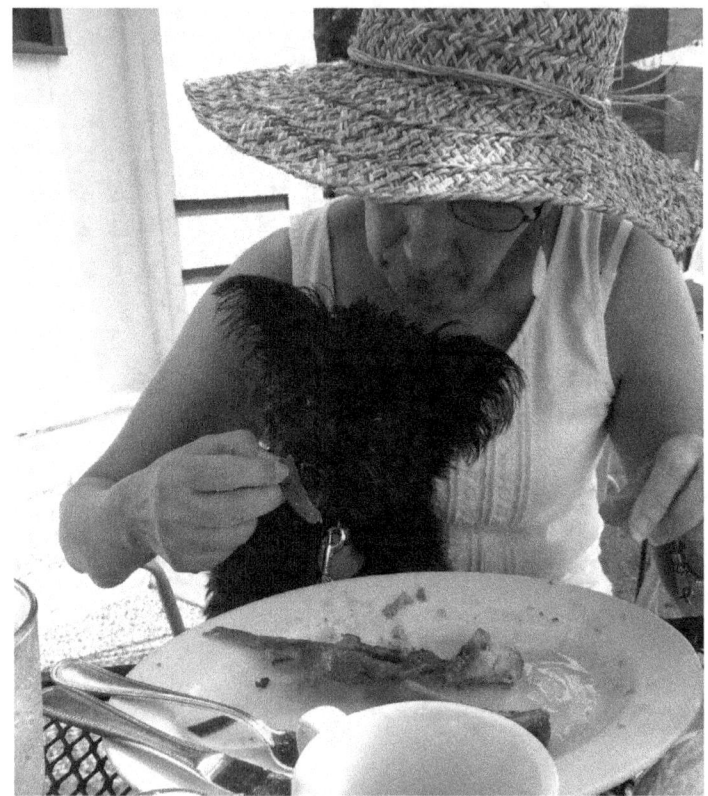

Eddie enjoying his bacon breakfast with us at City Square Café.

CHAPTER 6

Chapter 6: The Heart Transplant

At the hospital, Terry got settled in the hospital bed and I tried to get comfortable in a straight back lounge chair. We started watching TV, but she was so excited. She was like a little kid in a candy store with a pocketful of money. Finally, I said, "Please go to sleep. Tomorrow is going to be a long day and you need to be rested."

Around 3 a.m. on Wednesday, July 27, the anesthesiologist came to get her signature on the consent forms. He then reviewed the procedure and reminded her she could wake up and not be transplanted. Call it false labor, if you prefer, but the technical term they use is "dry run." He explained that if the surgeon finds something wrong with the new organ, or has any other reservations, he will not go forward with the transplant operation.

The anesthesiologist then administered some sedatives to relax her and help her to sleep. Even with the sedatives, she was still bouncing around. At 4 a.m., she got up and went to the bathroom. When she came out, she was dancing around the room. She came over to my chair and started kissing me. "I'm going to be normal again! We will be able to do normal things! Oh, how wonderful it will be!" she said.

I said, "Please, will you go to bed? Did that doctor make a mistake and give you uppers instead of the sedatives? It's hard enough to get any sleep in this chair without you crawling all over me." She finally took the hint and went to bed. Or it could have been that I told her I would take the bed and she could have the chair if she didn't settle down. Honestly, I'm not sure which one it was.

At 5:15 a.m., Terry's nurse came in, woke her up, and handed her a bottle of antibacterial soap and instructed her to shower, washing her whole body twice with the soap, and paying special attention to scrubbing from her neck to her abdomen. At 5:55 a.m., a technician arrived with the gurney to take her down to pre-op. We arrived there a few minutes later. Once there, I realized she was waiting in the same cubicle she was in for the LVAD surgery. I told her that was a good sign. Our daughter Kelly arrived a few minutes later. We were asked to wait in the family waiting area. Once I sat down, I realized this was the same chair I was in while I waited during the LVAD surgery. It allowed me the perfect vantage point to see her cubicle. The surgical prep started. On the wall I noticed a modified sort of clipboard. It was red on one side and green on the other. Each line printed on clear Plexiglas represented a progressive step in the pre-op that needed to be completed. The steps started on the left or red-colored half. As each step was completed the Plexiglas was slid to the green half. When all the steps where completed and in the green, they doubled checked everything again – just like I do in carpentry: measure twice, cut once.

The nurses started her intravenous (IV) line, reviewed her medical history and any allergies. The anesthesiologist, nurse anesthetist, operating room nurse and surgeon all came in and each did their necessary pre-op procedure to have Terry ready for the surgery.

While we were in the waiting area we met a woman named Dorothy whose sister was in the cubicle next to Terry. We learned that her sister was there for lung transplants and together surmised that both the heart and lungs were coming from the same donor. Later, I unofficially found out this was the case. Two lives in this hospital were about to be saved, one white, one black, because this person took the time to check "organ donor" on the driver's license application, or a family chose to donate a loved one's organs, giving life to others at their time of their sorrow.

Shortly after 7:15 a.m., Kelly and I were allowed to go back into her cubicle. The pre-op was completed, and now we just had to wait. Medication was administered into the IV to make Terry feel relaxed, but you wouldn't know it. She was ecstatic and raring to go. As members of the surgical team came to get her we both kissed her goodbye.

"Bring her back safe," I told the operating room nurse.

He replied, "We will treat her as if she is our own mother."

Even at the direst moments of my life, wit shines through. "I hope you really love your mother," was my final comment to the nurse.

They rolled my wife into the operating room at 8:03

Joseph Geraci

a.m.

We were told the surgery would last on average four to five hours. Kelly and I went to the family waiting room upstairs to wait. After six hours with no word, we were getting antsy. After seven hours, I was becoming a basket case and couldn't wait any longer. So buzzed the ICU and asked the nurse for help. Several minutes later, she came out with a cell phone in hand. One of the operating room nurses was on the line. I think her name was Jennifer, but I could be wrong. My brain was functioning on three brain cells at that point. You see, except for cat naps in a chair the night before, I had been up for 37 hours. Jennifer told me the new heart was in and working beautifully. Terry was off the bypass machine. They did have some bleeding that they needed to stop, and some repair work to do. She should be out in about two hours.

Almost four hours later, shortly after 7:30 p.m. the surgeon, Dr. Eric Sarin, came out to meet with us. We went into one of the family consultation rooms. We learned the full scope of the surgery. First off, the new heart was doing great, but because of the blood thinners she was on, they had trouble stopping the hemorrhaging. The body had treated the implantable cardioverter-defibrillator (ICD) and the left ventricular assist device (LVAD) as foreign objects and encrusted them with scar tissue. Also, due her small body cavity, her organs grew around the LVAD's pump and hoses. The pump and hoses had to be cut out. Due to the hemorrhaging, they needed to keep pumping in donated blood and fluids. As a consequence, they could not close her chest and induced a coma.

Kelly and I looked at each other in shock. "Her chest is

97

open?!" I said. "How can you leave her body open? Is she bleeding now? What about infection?" These were only a few of the questions I was spitting out, one after another, in such rapid fire sequence, I wasn't even giving him a chance to answer. He stopped me, and said he would answer my questions one by one to remove the fear and anxiety we had, and to reassure us that open-chest management is an effective and safe measure for someone in Terry's condition after heart transplant.

Dr. Sarin explained that her chest was sealed in a sterile, surgical bandage. The bandage was filled with an antibacterial solution that prevents infection and keeps the wound moist. Blood vessels were cauterized and the edges of the bone and muscles were covered with a wax for protection. She was receiving a controlled dose of an anesthetic, so she was not in any pain and her body was resting. As a result of all the fluids, it would not be safe to close her chest. That would exert too much pressure on the heart, preventing it from pumping. This procedure is used a lot in LVAD patients, he said. He went on to say they could leave her chest open for 30 days if needed, but he hoped they would be able to close on Sunday. This meant her chest would be open for five days! As much as I wanted to believe everything he said, I recognized that "doctor's poker face" I told you about back in the beginning of our journey. Dr. Sarin wore it. He said we could see her as soon as she was situated in the ICU. Finally, around 8:45 p.m., we were allowed in.

Kelly and I thought we were prepared, remembering how bad she looked after the LVAD surgery. This time seeing her scared the hell out of both of us. Kelly took one look at her and immediately ran out of the room, crying. I looked at this mass in the bed and said to myself, "This can't be my wife." Except for her hair, I didn't recognize her. Her head was the size of a basketball; her ears were each the size of softballs. Her eyes bulged out like two golf balls glued to the basketball. She had two holes where a nose should have been. She literally looked like a Macy's day balloon strapped to the bed. I never realized a human body had the capacity to expand that much. Even a sponge reaches its limit. I spoke to her ICU nurse. Terry was in critical but stable condition, and the next 72 hours would tell. I proceeded out into the hallway to comfort Kelly. She was standing out there, crying. I noticed she would try to peek at her mom, but when she saw her, she would just turn away and sob harder. I hugged her and said, "It's okay. Let's go home and get some rest. It has been a long day."

We left and headed home, in our separate cars, back to Manassas. On the way home, I stopped at a 7-Eleven convenience store to grab a hot dog and coffee. When I walked into the house at 10 p.m., the phone was ringing. The call was from Kelly. She was frantic.

"DAD, where are you? Why didn't you answer the phone when the hospital called?" she said.

"I just walked in the door. My phone was on vibrate and I didn't feel or hear it. Why? What's going on?" I asked.

"They rushed Mom back into surgery. They couldn't control the hemorrhaging. Her blood pressure dropped. Get here ASAP," she said.

At 10:31 p.m. I was walking back into the ICU unit at Fairfax Hospital. One thing about these transplant centers is, there is always a surgical team on hand 24/7 not only for transplants, but to handle just such emergencies.

An hour and a half later, shortly after midnight, Kelly and I met with Dr. Anthony Rongione for an update. He told us all the bleeding was under control. There would still be some bleeding into the drain lines, but that was normal and not to worry. He said to remember that the level of blood thinners she had been on really slowed the clotting process. Now, with all the blood products she'd received, it flushed the thinners out of her body and she was beginning to clot normally.

I remained at the hospital and talked periodically to her nurse, Theresa, who stayed in Terry's room with her throughout the night, monitoring her. I was curious as to how much fluid they pumped inside her. Theresa said, with the transplant surgery, she had received 19 pints of donated blood, plus four more pints during the second surgery to stop the bleeding, for a total of 23 pints of blood, 16 pints of platelets, and 18 pints of plasma. She received grand total of 56 pints of donated blood products, or 26 quarts or 7 gallons. Plus, she was given a number of units of saline solution but I did not know how much. Keep in mind, you only have 13 pints of blood to begin with. Wow! I sat there for a few minutes to digest all this, literally numb. I finally left the hospital at 2 a.m. and made it home just before 3 a.m. I went upstairs to bed. At this point, I had been up for almost 47 hours and thought to myself, when this is over and the adrenaline stops I'll probably crash for a month. I dosed off around 4 a.m.

The final total of all the blood products Terry would receive was 29 pints of blood, 24 pints of platelets and 18 pints of plasma. I never did get a final total on the number of bags of saline she received.

One final note, from this point on, you may notice a little different approach to the way I tell our story. Allow me to explain: this whole book is taken from my notes, my journals, my email updates and from my memory. When our journey started, I would write things down sporadically, sometimes weeks after the event. By the time we reached the transplant, Terry had quite a following of people concerned for her progress and wanting updates. So I was writing journal entries in real time as the events occurred. That way, when I started sending out email updates to friends and family, they were experiencing it as if they were watching the "News at 11."

However, at the time of the transplant, things went into turbo drive. I knew I could never keep up. Word started filtering out that she had the transplant. At home, there were a number of phone messages asking about her. I changed our answering machine message to say, "If you want information on Terry, leave your email and I will add you to the list." Before I knew it, the list had grown to more than 100 people.

I started calling the days "Heart + number of days"; it just seemed easier to title the subject line of the emails in this way. I put a postscript in one of the early emails, promising not to make them a daily occurrence.

The support I received from all these people was unbelievable. They all encouraged me to update daily, hourly or whenever I could. As much as writing these updates helped me, they seemed to have the same positive effect on the recipients. I have included many of the responses we received from these wonderful people after each Heart + update. I know without their support and prayers I never would have it through this ordeal. These people and the Lord have been my strength throughout these trying times.

Here are a few responses to the Heart + updates.

I will keep my fingers crossed and send you all my best wishes. I know how difficult yet hopeful this period must be as my brother had two open heart surgeries and is now doing very well. My thoughts are with you and your wife.

I have added her to the prayer list at Mclean Bible Church. Please keep us informed on her progress and how you are doing. I know that the caregiver is the last person that others think of during these trying times.

Please let me know if there is anything I can do to help!! OOO XXX

I just wanted you to know you and Terry are in my prayers for a speedy recovery. Hang in there.

Happy with Terry's good progress, stay strong in this difficult time.

We will continue to keep you and Terry in prayer. God Bless you my friend. If there is anything else we can do, please don't hesitate to call. God Bless you both!

If she needs more blood I am a donor and have B Positive if that helps.

I am so thankful for her new heart and I am sure you are overwhelmed with everything that is going on…please know you are in my thoughts and prayers. When this is all over I, and I am sure the rest of the group, would love for you to bring Terry to the meeting so we can meet her.

We are praying and thinking of you all Uncle Joe!

That's great news to hear she is stabilized. We can only imagine how difficult it's been for you both, as well as the rest of the family. Please know we send our love and well wishes to all of you and especially to Terry as she continues to fight her way through the process. Keep us posted on her progress, and hopefully more good news that she will be coming home soon.

We're all so glad she got a donor heart and all is well. I'm sure it's a big relief for you. I know she has a long road to recovery but at least the worse is over. God Bless modern medicine!

CHAPTER 7

Part Three: Post Transplant

Chapter 7: The Intensive Care Unit

Thursday, July 28 – Heart + 1 – I woke up, showered and dressed. I seemed to be in the movie *Groundhog Day*. I was reliving the previous day over and over in my mind. Finally, I made it downstairs, brewed some coffee and sent out the first Heart + 1 email update. As I sat there, holding a cup of coffee, I was trying to make sense of what was happening. Little did I know at the time, this was to be one of the strangest days of my life. Later, as I backed out of the driveway, the CD player picked up where it left off, playing Neil Diamond's Greatest Hits CD. The song was *"I've Been This Way Before,"* one of Terry's favorites. That's all it took. I just broke down and started crying. I cried almost the entire 25 miles to the hospital. I can't give a specific reason why. My best guess it was a combination of stress, fear, anxiety, lack of sleep and helplessness. Or, perhaps it stemmed from last night. Growing up, Dad taught my brothers and I that a man loves, protects and defends his family at all costs. Last night, seeing her there in a coma, I felt totally worthless as a man. Here was the woman I have loved and cherished, my best friend, and I could do absolutely nothing to help her.

As I was driving to the hospital, our friend, Susanna Barolin, the co-owner of City Square Café in Manassas with her husband, Chef Robert, called me on my cell phone. Her words of encouragement and her positive thoughts at the exact point when I was feeling my lowest, lifted my spirits tremendously. As we talked, she helped me to calm down, take a deep breath and relax. She was very concerned about my safety and getting to the hospital in one piece. I made it okay, parked in the parking garage and went up to the ICU. Before I could enter her room, I had to wash my hands thoroughly and use antibacterial spray. Terry was what the medical professionals called "transplant hot" – she was pumped so full of anti-rejection drugs that her immune system was severely compromised. Any exposure to germs, resulting in infection, could prove fatal.

Terry's nurse gave me an update on her condition. Later, I found out the doctors were surprised she made it through the night. Hearing them say that depressed me even more. So I settled into the chair and decided to read emails. I needed a laugh, so I opened some. I knew I would find some jokes in there and perhaps they would cheer me up. I opened several from my brother, Augie, and got a good chuckle. Then I noticed one from Carol D., a friend in the business networking group of which I am a member. In it, she said, *Joe, heard about your wife and will pray for her. Oh my, let me pray right now.* She typed the following prayer into the email.

"Gracious Heavenly Father, we praise you for the heart that is working and acknowledge you as our source of life and very good and perfect gift. We ask for your grace and healing touch for the swelling to go down and that everything will function / work right when she comes out of the coma. We ask for a hedge around her to protect her from staph infections and that she will have a speedy healing. We ask for strength and peace for Joe. We ask in Jesus' name, Amen."[3]

As I read this prayer, I felt a pressure on my left shoulder as if there was a hand on it, giving me a comfort and reassurance I cannot really express in words. I experienced a total peace and a calmness, as if to say, "Don't worry. She will be okay." All the weight of the world was lifted off my shoulders. My spirits changed, I felt great and knew from that moment on, Terry would be okay. It would not happen tomorrow, but she will have a full recovery.

I had a similar experience only one other time in my life, in July 2000. My oldest brother, Sal, passed away and I wrote his eulogy. With each rewrite, I attempted to read it aloud and I couldn't make it through. I was so emotional as I read it, my lips moved but no words came out. I was worried I would do this in front of a church full of people.

I was a nervous wreck sitting in the pew. I was afraid of dishonoring my brother. When the time came to walk up to the pulpit to speak, I got up and started across the chancel area at the front of the altar. I thought my knees were going to buckle if not then, for sure, when I climbed the steps of the pulpit. However; as I was ready to begin, I felt the presence of my brother Sal and my dad next to me. I read the eulogy flawlessly. This was the only time I was ever able to do this. Even today, 12 years later, I cannot read the copy of his eulogy, which hangs in our foyer, without choking up.

Several minutes after reading Carol's prayer, Father Charles Merkle III, the Catholic chaplain for Inova Fairfax Hospital, came in. We chatted for a couple of minutes and then he administered the Prayers of the Sick and the Anointing of the Sick. I received communion for her since she was unable to receive. For those of you who are not familiar with the Catholic religion, communion is a wafer which is consecrated during the Mass and represents the body of Jesus. This practice was first performed by Jesus at the last supper with his disciples.

Afterwards in chitchatting with him, I discovered he was a railfan. The common interest both comforted and distracted me as we talked about his favorite railroad, the Baltimore and Ohio (B&O).

I can't explain how I felt for the rest of the day. If I tried, you would think I'm crazy. (For those who know me, you already think that). As the day progressed, Terry showed small improvements. Her oxygen level was up. Her blood sugar numbers were great. Her kidneys and liver functions were normal. The swelling was going down. Her condition was classified as critical but stable, so much so, they scheduled her back to operating room the next day, Friday, July 29. On the way home that evening, I was driving west on Braddock Road and observing a beautiful orange sunset. I found myself crying again. This time, they were tears of joy. For the first time in this whole four and half year ordeal, I really can see the light at the end of the tunnel. I felt for the first time today, everything was finally going to be okay!

Heart + 1 Responses:

I can't tell you how much this story means to me. What a wonderful way to close out the day, reading your beautiful testimony of faithful love of our Lord Jesus. It's truly amazing how the Lord uses the body of Christ to minister to each other. For Him to give you that special touch on your shoulder is so, so precious. You're not crazy at all; on the contrary, you are well loved by the Lord and you know it and want to tell the world! I encourage you to do so, like you did tonight. Don't let the enemy talk you out of it. Thank you again, Joe, for opening your heart and in doing so, revealing the Lord's heart for all others to see. Little do you know how your story will minister to someone else in their hour of need. Sleep well my friend, in the loving arms of our Lord who cares for you.

God Bless Terry, you and your family.

I'm glad to hear Terry is showing progress. I can't speak for everyone, but feel free to write as often as you would like. It helps to keep you strong and deal with the roller coaster ride you are on.

Knowing Terry these past 44 years, I always knew she was a calm, cool and tough Little S---! Squeeze her hand for us.

Wow – can't say much to that other than I feel Him from time to time especially when I need Him the most.

Laura forwarded me the email update you sent regarding Terry. I am so happy for all of you regarding the positive gains and progress that Terry has shown! It is difficult to remember at times. Talk soon.

We are keeping you and Terry in our prayers. Thank you so much for the updates. We are in the Midwest right now, so please keep us informed.

When you are with Terry and you are monitoring her care, you make a difference. Just observing and trying to understand the care she receives makes a difference to the doctors and nurses. I spent a couple of months, almost every day, at my mom's side when she had a stroke. Had I not been paying attention, the actions of one of the techs would have led to my mom receiving an unnecessary surgical procedure. Our doctors and nurses who are giving the care are competent and caring – but none will care as much as family. Seeing your compassion and concern for your wife, increases theirs. I know what you mean – the sun sets every day, but some days it lets us reflect on our lives and even big tough Italian guys get choked up.

Joe, while I haven't walked in your shoes, I have nothing but the best wishes, thoughts and prayers for both of you. Terry needs this chance. She beat cancer and it left a bad scar. Let's look at it a bit differently. Someone had to die to give her life. There is more than two of you involved in this. God works in the absolutely most mysterious ways, far beyond practical and normal. This also brings out your friends and the healing. I believe the surgeons and staff working with

109

the heart to make it work to get Terry back have the same hopes we all have. The family who made this gift possible is right there with you both. God smiles and will do whatever His will is. These tests are horribly hard and take a toll on everyone, but if all goes well, all these efforts, it is worth every tear, every prayer and thank you from all who are involved. It is amazing how at these times we all feel that we can control things and don't really rely on others but when the chips are down and we're at our weakest – we can become our strongest, no matter what, because of others who step forward in times of need and times of crisis. Don't hide your tears, Joe, for I sincerely hope when Terry opens her eyes again and speaks your name the world will be all right again. Remember you're not alone.

P.S. – Don't stop the updates. It's therapy for all of us. If you need platelets, I can donate. Call if you do.

Joe, you can send updates whenever you want – daily, hourly or whenever. We all love you and Terry and love to get the updates. It helps us to know how Terry is doing (and you as well) and to know especially what to pray for. God bless you and give you strength.

Thank you for sharing your story. I really do believe there is a Higher Power at work; we are not alone in this world. I felt it many times when my husband was ill and it was a comfort.

We will continue to pray that the swelling will continue to go down. It is awesome it went down that much that they scheduled her. Just a little more…. Praise God that she is doing well. I know the hours seem so long and it's hard to wait. My son had open heart surgery and they had to keep him asleep because they thought they damaged his esophagus with a tube. They brought in a specialist to investigate. They kept my son asleep until everything could be worked out. It was hard. Keep me posted.

You are a wonderful person and you are most certainly Terry's biggest treasure. I look forward to hearing your updates on Terry. We are all anxious to receive news from you.

I thank God for putting the words of encouragement and the phone call you needed – His timing is always perfect! Keep leaning on Him as the rest of us lift you and Terry through this. Looking forward to your next update!

Thank you so much for including me in your emails regarding your wife's progress with the heart transplant. My thoughts and prayers are with you and your bride as you make your way through this challenging ordeal. At this point you need to trust in the goodness of the Lord above and in the competence of the professionals that you've retained to perform the operation. Please keep me in the loop regarding her progress and also in how you're doing in dealing with the realty of the situation. I wish you all the best and will continue to include both of you in my prayers. Best Always.

Friday, July 29 – Heart + 2 – I arrived late, around 11 a.m. Terry was scheduled to go back into surgery around noon. On my way to the hospital I received a call from the kidney doctor and the anesthesiologist. They both needed consent forms signed. The request from the kidney doctor was surprising. He informed me it was a precaution in the event her kidneys crashed, so they could start her on dialysis immediately. Her kidneys were in overdrive to remove all the fluids; hopefully, they would continue to handle it. If not, they had to be prepared in the event of an emergency. She was rolled into surgery at 12:50 p.m. To move her was quite an operation. They had to take all the equipment with her. This included the bed, three IV poles with 18 IVs, the heart monitoring equipment, and all the drain lines and their collection receptors, plus the ventilator machine. As Terry and her entourage rolled by, they looked like an outlandish float in a parade. Surgery took two hours. She was back in her room in the ICU at 3:15 p.m. I spoke to Dr. Sarin and he assured me everything was okay. The heart is doing great, no infection, they cleaned the incision and applied a new dressing. Everything was good. She was still too swollen to close her chest. They would try again on Sunday, July 31.

Heart + 2 Responses:

Glad this next chapter in your wife's road to better health has happened. You do what you need to get her back on her feet. Our thoughts are with you both.

I'm so glad to hear Terry finally got the transplant. I'm praying for her and I will add her to my church prayer list. Let me know if I can do anything for you and when she can have visitors. I would love to come.

Tina and I think this fabulous news!

I was delighted to hear about wife's transplant! I hope the swelling comes down soon. Sending lots of good vibes and hugs your way.

My very best to you and your wife. My prayers and thoughts are with you both as she braves the transplant and you hold it all together. Please add me to your update list.

I will keep praying for Terry. God will look after her.

Saturday, July 30 – Heart + 3 – Terry had a very peaceful night. The heart, liver and kidneys were all functioning beautifully. The ICU nurses and the kidney specialist were still monitoring the kidneys very closely. With the medication she is receiving, her kidneys are still working in overdrive. Her face is almost back to normal and so are her ears. Her hands and fingers are still really swollen. They removed one more IV drip. Another good sign, she is now down to 15 IVs from the 21 with which they started. Plus, she has not needed any additional blood products for two days now. The new heart is working wonderfully; today the output ranged from 4.9 to 5.1 liters of blood per minute and a squeeze rate of 3.2. A year ago, her heart's output was only 1.2 to 1.7 liters per minute. Her color is back and doesn't look pale any more. The plan is still to attempt closing her up tomorrow. Every day has been getting better. My fears and apprehensions have all but disappeared. Ever since last Thursday [July 28] I am at peace with this whole ordeal. I really can't explain it, but two friends explain this way: The first said I was touched by the hand of God. I don't feel worthy of that honor. I'm one of those who go with "Lord I am not worthy say but the word and my soul shall be healed."[4] The second said it was the Holy Spirit bestowing his grace and strength. Again, I can't agree with that because of what I just stated. I will go along believing I was touched by an Angel sent by the Lord. I like to think the Good Lord gave her this new heart so his ears would stop ringing and he could once again have a little peace in heaven.

Courtney is her nurse today. She is from Texas, but more importantly she and her husband are train buffs. All of the ICU nurses Terry has had have been super, but Courtney is my favorite. I play 20 questions with her five times over. Many of these may be classified in the stupid question department; however, she takes the time to explain what each of the drips or IVs do or why Terry's blood sugar has to be tested hourly even though she is not diabetic or what all indictors on the ventilator mean. She gives me a detailed education on Terry's dressing and how it works. She answers all my questions on the induced coma. Plus she encourages me to talk to Terry while she is in the coma. "Yours is a familiar voice and she recognizes your tone," she says.

"Here, watch," she adds, and I do. She has to clean Terry's mouth to help prevent infection. This is done about every four hours. It's very uncomfortable because of the ventilator tube going down her throat and she doesn't like it. Courtney starts the procedure. Terry is making faces and moving her mouth around. Courtney says, "Now hold her hand and just start talking to her." I did and she stopped with the faces and stopped fighting Courtney. After Courtney finished, I move the chair next to the bed and for the rest of the afternoon I held Terry's hand and just kept talking to her as if she is awake. I also run my hand through her hair sometimes. As I do this, I can see Terry's eyes move rapidly under her closed lids, as if she's in normal REM sleep.

[3] The Prayer of Humble Access is a prayer immediately prior to communion in Mass.

Heart + 3 Responses:

Thank you for this update Joe. I love how you love your wife and the Lord. Love is very healing. Blessings.

GREAT NEWS, JOE!

Glad to hear things are moving in a positive direction. She's a strong woman and will be back giving you a hard time real fast.

Wow I know Aunt Terry got a long way to recovery but from the sound of things she is getting better. You know I read the email before I went to church I started to cry happy tears. Please let me know when Aunt Terry gets a room please. Thank you. You know God does work in remarkable ways and God answers God hears and answers prayers. Aunt Terry you are in my thoughts and prayers Uncle Joe Nikki Sean Kelly Olivia all of you are in my thoughts and prayers too. I love you all more than any of you can realize. Love short, short little, little Lisa Boo Hoo I don't think I'll ever grow. Oh well there's

Miracle Grow Luck with that. Love Lisa [This one especially means a lot to me because it was written by my niece who is mentally challenged. I only corrected the misspelled words. I know that for her to write this paragraph is fantastic in my book. We love you, too, Lisa.]

We just returned from a beach vacation and had a wonderful time this week with one of our sons and his kids. But the most wonderful thing that has happened in the last week is the news you've sent about Terry's operation and the truly miraculous response to the transplant. Praise God from whom all blessings flow.

I'm so glad to hear Terry is doing well. I had my church pray for her today and put her on the continued prayer list. I also had my sister put her on her church prayer list in Maryland and my cousin in New York, who works at the church rectory, will add her to their list, too. I'm looking forward to Terry busting your chops again. Somebody needs to keep you in line. Please let me if you need anything. I'm just 20 minutes from Fairfax Hospital and will be glad to help with anything you need. Take care of yourself and Terry.

Hi Joe, I would like to make something for Terry. Can you tell me the color of her favorite chair or couch, if that's where she likes to relax? Thanks.

Joe, hang in there. Terry is not in an emergency situation so that is good. She is doing so well and improving steadily. Gracious Heavenly Father, whose grace and mercy flows every day, we thank you that Terry is doing so well and that your steady hand is upon her. We pray that Terry will go to the operating room at just the right time, YOUR time, and that you will guide everyone in the operating room to a successful and miraculous closing of her chest. We thank you for the life you have given her and for her faithful husband. We ask your blessing upon them at their hour of need so that Joe can feel the peace that passes all understanding, a peace that only you can give. In Jesus' name we pray, Jesus, the name that is above all names, Jesus

115

the highest ruler with authority over every other power. We thank you and praise you. Amen.

Sunday, July 31 – Heart + 4 – Improvement continues. The doctors removed some more of her meds and her ICU nurse washed her hair this morning. I brought in her brush to comb it. Courtney is back on duty today and of course I had my list of 20 questions. The doctors couldn't bring her into the operating room today only because, between transplants and emergencies, none were available. Her doctors ordered the start of intravenous feeding for her today since she did not go into surgery. A tube was inserted through her nose. The feeding will go on until midnight. Later today, the staff will change her linens and check her back for bedsores and pooled blood. Watching them do this while she is in the bed is quite interesting. They bring in a whole crew of nurses and technicians and carefully roll her on her side to make half the bed. Then they put her on her back and roll her on her other side to make the other half. The beds in the ICU are unbelievable. The mattresses inflate and deflate with air in a rhythmic movement to prevent bed scores. The mattress and bed can expand lengthwise to eight feet or they can reduce it to fit the patient. Plus it has every feature imaginable that you can think of and then some.

My brother, Augie, and my niece, Jessica, came down from Buffalo to help out yesterday. With them here I don't have to worry about the house or cooking. I left early today as our daughter Nikki is coming in tonight.

Heart + 4 Responses:

Will say a prayer that all goes well and she gets to the OR today so she can start her way back to consciousness.

I'm so happy to hear Terry is continuing to do so well. I'm going to save your email about your voice having a calming effect and when Terry starts coming to shows again, I'll share it with her as a reminder, especially as you're setting up and breaking down.

Keep me posted as she is coming out of the coma so I know how to pray.

Joe, you're wonderful! I was in a drug-induced coma when I had an accident in 1999. She can recognize your voice and she may remember some of what she hears. I know I did. She may also hear what the doctors say so don't let her hear anything scary or negative. Please let me know me know if there is anything I can help with.

Hi, what time are you coming home tonight? I have a nice roast in the crock pot with potatoes and carrots if you want to swing by and grab a bite before going home. I know it may be late and that's okay.

Monday, August 1 – Heart + 5 – WHAT A GREAT DAY! Terry went into the operating room today so the surgeon could close her chest. I met her anesthesiologist. His name is Dr. Micquel and is really a cool guy. I asked him about the coma. If all went well, how long it would take for her to come out of the coma? He replied, "It could take as little as four hours or as many as five days." I also met a surgical nurse who was part of the medical team that went to procure the organ. This surgical nurse was also in the OR the first night when Terry was taken back into surgery to stop the hemorrhaging. She was so happy Terry was doing well; she said to me, "Terry really gave them one hell of a scare that night!" After they took her in, I left the ICU unit. The staff didn't like you in the empty room because when she is brought back it takes a while to settle her in.

Now picture the hospital as an "H" lying on its back. The rooms are on the vertical legs of the H and horizontal leg connects the wings. The horizontal leg has the family waiting rooms and restrooms along a long corridor where they park spare equipment. This corridor has one side with huge windows. Whenever I cannot be in her room, I pull the blind in her room way up before I leave. Then I go to the corridor and grab one of the chairs and line it up so I can see into her room. It was comforting for me to keep an eye on her this way.

I sat there and waited. After they brought her back and Dr. Micquel found me. He asked, "Why are you sitting in the corridor?"

I replied, "I have a bird's eye view of her room."

He laughed and told me her chest was closed and there was no infection. Doctor Sarin would be out as soon as he could to give me a full report. I did not care; I already heard the two things I wanted to hear. I continued sitting there, watching her room.

Several hours passed. Dr. Micquel walked by and asked, "What are you still doing here?"

I said, "Waiting for them to let me back in."

He motioned for me to wait and proceeded into the ICU. Next thing I saw was Dr. Micquel in the window of Terry's room with her nurse, Ruppa, under his arm, pointing at me. I could read his lips telling her to wave me in, which she did. When I got to her room we all had a good laugh and he went on his way.

I stayed until 7 p.m. with Terry and then I went home. My brother Augie had dinner ready for me. After we ate, it was time to celebrate. In 1990, I bought a fifth of 15-year-old single malt scotch to save for celebrating the Buffalo Bills' first Super Bowl victory. As you can guess, that bottle was never opened. That is, until tonight. My brother Augie and I sat on the front porch, smoked two cigars and killed that bottle. What happened today with the success of Terry's heart transplant operation was better than any Super Bowl victory. While we sat drinking, my brother paid me a compliment that meant a lot to me. He said "Joe, you have been dealt a really poor hand. But you stepped up to the plate and have done a great job. Dad would be proud."

At the end of the Heart + 5 email update, I asked everyone on the email list to pray for the donor and her family. Our family was happy because of this gift of life. Their family was suffering over the loss of their loved one.

"I would like to UP that little request of yours by asking for people to just mark their driver's licenses as Organ Donors," replied a friend named Debbie. "The person who offers such a potential gift lives on in the recipient and the life they save may be one that saves the world!" After I made the request I was surprised by the number who already had signed the donor cards. Another eight to ten emailed they would do it. Still others volunteered to donate blood or blood platelets to help replenish the blood blank. All of these actions warmed our hearts.

Heart + 5 Responses:

So you asked we say a prayer for the donor and family and God to spread his Grace over her soul and for her family: Done, and a prayer to give you strength during this long and difficult process. I'm glad progress is being made.

What a wonderful celebration. Glad everything is moving forward. We will continue to keep prayers and thoughts going.

Hey Uncle Joe Aunt Terry I thought the beginning part was funny when I read it. Oh well anyway sounds like everything is going good on that end. So far so good one step at a time I know it's a lot of work if you could keep doing emails every day. I would really appreciate it a lot I will check them every day. I will also pray for Aunt Terry every morning and every night. I will also pray for the family who lost a loved one and their friends. I love you all very, very, very, very, very much love your niece Lisa

Thanks so much for the uplifting update. You'll have so much to tell Terry when she wakes up.

Awesome news…God is good!

That's Great Joe! P.S. – Hope you didn't have a hangover.

God is good indeed and this just shows us HE is totally in charge of our lives every day. Also prayer is the most powerful weapon we have. I'm praying for Terry and you, your family and for the family of the person whose heart is beating strong in Terry's chest. Talk about "no greater love."

That's great news. Shows the power of prayer! I had my church pray not only for Terry but; her donor on Sunday. If you ever find out who it was, I know they usually don't tell you, could you please let me know so I can make her mom a prayer shawl. Still praying.

GREAT NEWS! Keep up the good work! Sherry and I really appreciate being on the email list so we can follow Terry's progress and stay in touch with you as you cheer her on. We will most certainly pray for the donor and her family. In a day or so you will receive a gift certificate for Silver Diner. At some point you might like to grab some grub coming or going from the hospital.

Thank you so much. Tina has been sharing the updates with me. I'm so glad that things are progressing so well. I am keeping you both in my prayers and the woman's family whose donation made this all possible.

This message just makes me smile and Rejoice in the Lord! Blessings to you and your family!

GREAT NEWS, JOE! So happy to hear she's progressing so well. God is not ready to take her for a long, long time. We will keep her in our prayers until she is fully recovered, then an extra prayer to God thanking him for bringing her to that point. You know of course, if you need anything all you have to do is let me know. Love you both.

I was so happy to get your email and even happier to hear of Terry's progress. I'm glad your brother was there to celebrate this milestone with you. Our prayers are with you by the minute and we are also remembering the family of the person whose life was lost but who gave such an amazing gift. I wish I were closer to offer more help, but the kids and I are in Erie till the 21st. Please don't forget to take care of yourself, too, Joe. Terry is very blessed to have you and will no doubt be looking for you first when she regains consciousness. You have a whole lot of love and prayers being sent to you and it will continue. For now, God is good and we give our thanks and praise to Him. I will keep in touch and please whisper to my friend that I love her and can't wait to see her. Boy, won't we have a lot to chat about.

Celebrating with you (not in drink) but with praises!

The family that is grieving right now, I hope they know what a blessing their loved ones heart gave to someone else, just by the choice of being a donor...I will be praying for that family as well.

Tuesday, August 2 – Heart + 6 – The doctor cut off the drugs that were inducing Terry's coma at 5 a.m. Now we just have to sit and wait for her to come back to us. I stayed next to the bed and talked to her. I was really hoping she'd wake up in the four-hour window the doctor said would be the minimum time. After being there all day, the best I got was more eye and foot movement. A couple times she looked like she would open her eyes, but then again that could have been wishful thinking on my part.

Today is support group day and the topic is transplants.

The guest speakers are previous transplant recipients. They will each speak about the healing and life after transplant. This is the first time our daughters Kelly and Nikki have attended one of the support group meetings and this month's topic is perfect. After listening to the speakers, they were given the chance to ask them specific questions that related to their concerns about their mom. What Terry was experiencing was not that different from some of the other transplanted LVAD patients. Listening to them reinforced the fact that LVAD patients do have a more difficult time. Both Kelly and Nikki came away feeling better and more optimistic as well. They also learned firsthand a little more on how the transplant procurement process works. Allow me to share with you some of what I know.

The United Network of Organ Sharing (UNOS) is an organization contracted by the Federal government to provide for the fair distribution of donated organs. Our local group, the Washington Regional Transplant Community (WRTC) is tasked with following all the standards and policies established by UNOS. WRTC is responsible for working with the donor, the donor's family and for coordinating the procurement of the organs. Both the donor's family and the recipient's family have complete privacy. Neither family has any contact with the other unless both sides agree. If we wished to send a letter to the family we can do so. We would write the letter and give it to the hospital social worker. She, in turn, would forward it to the WRTC. WRTC, in turn, will notify the donor family of the letter or the fact we wish to make contact. The donor family then can either accept or decline. The WRTC would hold the letter in the event the family changes their mind at a later date.

When you are placed on the list, so is all your medical information pertinent for transplant matching, such as blood type, antibodies, height, weight, age, sex, plus a number of other factors. I do not know, and to be honest with you, I do not care to know. Over the past five years I have learned more about medicine than I ever wanted to learn in five lifetimes. What I was really happy to learn was that the donor was as close a match as you can get with two total strangers.

Heart + 6 Responses:

Thanks for the update. It would be great if we could schedule a blood donation event. I think this would be a way for those of us who feel the need to do something, to help.

We will keep you in our prayers. Our family has signed the donor cards. When you have a loved one who has had a transplant, it brings the importance of being a donor home. On the reverse side; when you lose a loved one, it is comforting to know they have helped someone else lead a better life. We've seen both sides.

GO TERRY! Thank you for the info. I'm sooo happy to know that she raised her eyebrows to you. Most times that would have been annoying, but today it's a blessing. You go get some more raised eyebrows today. Take care of yourself.

Again, please tell her we are thinking about her and praying for her. Hope today is a better day for response. Just this morning I was thinking about the fact I already marked my license to be an organ donor and now I know why. I always knew it was a good thing to do for others, however; I never knew I would be close to someone who needed an organ. It makes it even clearer as to why it is such a generous and thoughtful thing to do. Love to all.

Joe, I have been praying for you and your wife. I hope she recovers quickly and all is well.

I hope everything is going well!! Keep me posted. In my prayers.

Thank you so much for all the updates and for encouraging blood and organ donations. Your ordeal is a wakeup call to us all.

Wednesday, August 3 – Heart + 7 – Wow, what a week. Sometimes I think it's been an eternity; other times it feels like just a couple of minutes. The snooze meds have been off for 27 hours. Today she is in and out; mostly out. She opens her eyes about halfway. For the anesthetic drugs to be filtered out of the body, they have to slow the kidneys down to a normal pace. These drugs take longer to be filtered by the kidneys. With her kidneys working at an accelerated pace it doesn't allow for them to be removed because the blood is passing through them too quickly. They can't just slam the brakes. The kidneys need to be slowed down gradually to prevent any damage.

One time I asked her if she knew where she was. She nodded yes. This made the girls and me very happy. She continues to take baby steps and is moving forward. We're down to just six IVs from 21. In a twist on the venerable Timex watch slogan, I tell everyone that "Terry's my little Timex; she's taken a licking and keeps on ticking." Tomorrow hopefully she will be awake, and she better not complain she's tired.

Heart + 7 Responses:

Out of the more than 50 plus emails I receive overnight, yours is the first that I read. I'm glad that Terry is processing forward even though it feels like little itty bitty baby steps. Have a great day.

Every day the news is good! Prayers and love your way!

I love your humor in all of this. You and your family are an inspiration to me – still praying and so thankful for the positive prognosis!

GOD BLESS YOU TERRY and your family, wish we were

closer to you all. We'll keep you in our prayers.

We are so happy to know that she is coming back. We'll come to see her soon.

Hi Joe just heard the great news. I guess Terry is awake from her induced coma by now. Please let her know that I'm thinking of her. I really like your wife – she is a great down-to-earth lady with a twinkle in her eye. I suspect she was a ball of fire before all this happened. I just hope that you can keep up with her a year from now. Please keep me informed about her progress.

Thursday, August 4 – Heart + 8 – Today we start our second week. Well, it's official. My two remaining brain cells are dead. Yes, the adrenaline rush I've had for the last 10 days has subsided. This morning I tried to remember how long Terry's been in the hospital. I couldn't compute it in my head. So I had to use my fingers to count the days. Guess I will have to use my toes in two more days.

Terry is slowly waking up. She can open her eyes when you speak to her. She also seems to be aware of her surroundings. I told her Nikki was in town and would be here with Kelly later. She got this surprised look on her face and raised her eyebrows. Terry knew Nikki was coming down the first week of August. I figured she thought it is still July and something was wrong. I assured her everything was okay and I would explain everything later and answer her questions after the ventilator was out. Speaking of the ventilator, they lowered the settings to a rate of 8. This was done to start retraining her lungs to breathe on their own. Think of it as slapping a newborn on the behind. So far her lungs are responding. If they stop or slow down, the ventilator is preset to take over and prevent a problem. An alarm would sound to alert the staff.

Just to share a little antidote with you: Yesterday while waiting for the operating room team to come and take her for her first heart biopsy, an alarm went off down the hall. Virtually everyone – doctor, nurse and technician – in the ICU responded in seconds. I never did find out what happened, but I was comforted to witness how fast they responded to any emergency and to know Terry was surrounded by such excellently trained staff.

Terry went for her first heart biopsy/right heart catheterization today. What this does is measure all the pressures in the heart to see how well the heart is performing. While they are inside the heart they remove four scrapings from four different places to be analyzed. This test is how they determine if the new organ is being rejected. They will do the same test weekly for six weeks and then every other week until she reaches the three month mark. After that the tests will be monthly for six months, followed by once a quarter for up to one year. By knowing what her rejection level is, they can adjust her level of anti-rejection drugs. At transplant, she was given high levels of all the anti-rejection drugs. With each satisfactory biopsy, the dosage of the drugs is reduced. The idea is to reach the minimum amount of drugs necessary to prevent rejection. This, in turn, increases the patient's immune system and her ability to fight infections. It's quite a balancing act.

The Dragon Lady had to draw some blood today (guess they wanted some of the 29 pints back). I call her the Dragon Lady because she is a strict by-the-book, never-smile, kind of nurse, sort of like a Marine drill sergeant. Please do not misunderstand me; she's an excellent nurse

– just really, really, really strict. She even wanted me to disinfect my lips before I kissed Terry on the forehead. As she began to draw blood, Terry's blood pressure spiked. The Dragon Lady said, "Terry's getting excited."

So I said, "Terry, this is no time to get hot and bothered."

I thought the Dragon Lady would pee her pants she laughed so hard.

I know this has been a lengthy update but there is one more thing I would like to share. For the six of you who have either called or emailed me saying you already have signed the donor cards, or have been so touched by Terry's courage and faith through this ordeal that you have decided to become donors, on behalf of our entire family, we THANK YOU. Terry's life and the lives of all transplant patients would not have been saved without the generosity of the donors and their families.

Heart + 8 Responses:

Joe - keeping you both in our prayers.

This wonderful news!

What great news! We are so happy that Terry is doing so well!

I've been an organ donor for years – the problem is, my organs keep getting older. I hope that someone will be able to use something – to give the gift of life would be an amazing thing! God bless you both!

So glad too things are improving. You are such a hoot! "Hot and bothered." No wonder the nurse lost it. FYI I've been a donor since the first time they offered it years ago. I've always known of the great gift it is and I figured whatever they take I wasn't going to use anymore anyway. Sending you hugs.

Oh Joe! Thanks so much for letting me know! I'm so happy for both of you! Freddy was transplanted last week, and I saw Greg, the nice young man who came to meetings with his wife, was also transplanted! This makes my month! Thanks again, Joe and have a great day!

Great news about Terry's progress! I love your updates.

I'm also a donor — have been for years   and I will donate blood later in August when I return to Virginia. Replacing the volume used is a great idea.

Can't wait for her to get her milkshake!

Hi Joe, wonderful news about your wife, we had no idea. You and your family will be in our prayers, please keep us updated and God Bless!

Yep, I am already an organ donor and have been for years! Hang in there and hope my Maxine emails have given you a chuckle.

Thank you for reaching out to me, keeping me posted on Terry's condition and adding me to your email list. The last week sounded terrifying and I'm so glad she is making tremendous improvements since this past Monday. I'm planning on donating to a local blood bank on Terry's behalf given that I'm outside the area. Speak soon!

Went and gave platelets and red blood cells today for you guys. I'm so happy to hear Terry is doing so well.

Hi Joe, Just checking in to see how all is going with your wife (and you). I hope all is progressing positively. I'd like to let the folks in NVHG [Northern Virginia Handcrafters Guild] know how it's going at the meeting Monday.

Friday, August 5 – Heart + 9 – Things keep moving forward and the news continues to be positive. We received the results of the biopsy taken yesterday. Her rejection rate was a 1. Rejection rates are measured from 0 to 3. A transplant recipient will only get a 0 if the organ is from an identical twin; if not, a 1 is great. The worst is 3 and means severe or acute rejection for numerous reasons. Since she had a 1, the amount of anti-rejection drugs she is receiving will be lowered. This process will be repeated weekly for the next five weeks.

Terry's floating in and out. When she is awake, we can sort of talk to her, one way only. If she needs something you have to keep asking questions until you get the right answer. We both want the ventilator out. This can't happen until her lungs support themselves. Earlier they had the ventilator set at almost the lowest setting to see how her lungs performed. However her breathing rate kept spiking, meaning she was hyperventilating on the ventilator. The alarms sounded and the machine kicked in to take over and regulate the number of breathes per minute. Her lungs need more training. It is nice having her able to respond to me and know I'm there.

Terry's nurse today is Livia, and I'm really glad. Her nurse the past couple of days was The Dragon Lady. Livia had to change the dressing in Terry's mouth because she kept biting the inside of her cheeks raw. She absolutely hates this. It is extremely uncomfortable for her. Livia had to move the ventilator hose around and it really irritates her throat. Terri squeezed my hands while listening to Livia's commands. Kelly was rubbing her forehead and I was talking to her. I know she is still uncomfortable but now it's at least a little more bearable knowing we are here.

Saturday, August 6 – Heart + 10 – Wow, we reached the double digits today! Terry is semi-alert and trying to communicate. She went on another road trip today for a CAT scan. Terry has been badly bruised. Two days ago I inquired about it. Her right arm was black and blue as well as her palm and fingers. The only white in her hand were the lines. Plus the right side of her neck was also severely black and blue. They were not concerned then; today they are worried. They think she may to bleeding and want to check her out to be sure. She really wants to talk but can't with the ventilator tube in. We tried writing but with the lack of strength and the swelling in her hand and fingers, she couldn't. Next we made an alphabet chart and so she could point to the letters. That did not work either. By the time we get this figured out, she will off the ventilator.

They started the first phase test again to see if her lungs are capable to breathe on their own. If she passes, they move on to the second phase of the test. Both phase one and two are two hours each. If she passes both phases, out comes the ventilator tube.

While all this has been going on, I had a personal dilemma that needed to be resolved. I had entered an international photo competition earlier in the year. One of the train photos I entered was selected as one of 45 finalists out of more than 1,500 entries. The grand prize winners would be announced on Saturday in Fort Lauderdale, Florida. I had booked my flight back in June; now I had to decide whether to go or stay. The doctors said to go; that Terry was in good hands. I was torn whether to go or not go. Our daughters also told me to go; they would be there. In the end, I cancelled my reservations and stayed. If I won, they could mail me the prize.

The CAT scan taken earlier was negative. The bruising was a result of when they removed the implantable cardioverter-defibrillator (ICD) from her chest. It just didn't appear earlier. They also did an ultrasound test and found out she has a lot of blocked veins as a result of the breast cancer and radiation. We were told not to worry; the body has many redundant venial pathways in the body and her health would not be affected in any way.

Sunday, August 7 – Heart + 11 – I'm sorry there were no email updates for the last two days. I was wiped out when I came home Friday night and I went to bed. Last night, I stayed at the hospital until almost midnight.

Terry totally came out of the coma yesterday. This morning I called the hospital like I normally do at the beginning of each day to see how her night was. Her nurse Tracy said she was off the ventilator. Boy, was I excited. I told Tracy I was bringing Terry her chocolate milkshake and cinnamon bun. Terry made it very clear to me before the surgery that when she woke up she wanted two things: a chocolate milkshake from the Silver Diner and a cinnamon bun. I thought the nurse was going to come through the phone and choke me. After I arrived at the hospital I learned why. The ventilator stretched her vocal cords and her trachea had to learn to swallow again. They have to be careful that food particles do not get into her lungs. By the afternoon they had her sitting in a chair. Her voice was barely a whisper. We got our granddaughter Olivia in to see her for a couple of minutes and talk to her Granny. The visit did them both a lot of good. We had been telling Olivia all along that her Granny was doing well. To a 10-year-old though, seeing is believing. Olivia was so happy after seeing and talking to her Granny. She remained in the chair for several hours after they put Terry back in bed. A feeding tube was inserted through her nose. She was fed via the tube all night long. Tomorrow they will start to re-educate her trachea.

Heart + 11 Responses:

Fantastic! Give her a squeeze for us.

I can appreciate how tired you must be. All is good news.

You're doing a GREAT JOB! Wish we could be there. Feeling pretty helpless right now. Keep sending emails.

Baby steps! Glad to hear.

God Bless her!

That's great news and tremendous progress.

EXCELLENT!

Hey we New Yorkers have to stick together even if you are from the other New York and root for the Bills. Give her a big hug for me. I'm so glad she's off the ventilator.

Delighted to hear Terry's health is improving with her new heart. It's been quite an ordeal. The support of her family and friends has certainly helped pull you all through!

God Bless you both.

Wonderful news.

[I sent the first photo of Terry sitting up with the Heart +11 email update].

Beautiful.

Wow she looks great. Great news. Love and prayers.

I'm SOOO glad to see you sitting up.

You are beautiful! You look a lot better than I expected. You go girl!

Hi Joe, Mom and Dad moved to South Carolina. They love it. I am sharing printouts of your emails with Mom. They still have not set up their computer yet. Mom was thrilled to hear that Terry is awake and making progress. Please tell Terry Mom has been thinking of her and can't wait to see her. They will be back in September for a wedding.

What an inspiration! Please give her my very best along with a hug. Thank you, Joe for the updates.

My, My, What a blessing! Thank you Lord. We give you praise and glory for what you have done in Terry and Joe's life.

She's real fighter. Been thinking of you often.

My friend Charlie's son called to see how Terry was doing. He said he had swelling and was four days after transplant for follow up surgery. It will be two years next month since his heart transplant. He went home after three weeks.

Uncle Joe, Aunt Terry looks really great. When you see her tell Aunt Terry I said that Ok! Love and prayers Lisa

Wow! Incredible…continued thoughts and prayers! All the best.

YEAH TERRY!

Awesome! Please give her a hug for me. By the way I have been an organ donor on my driver's license for a long time.

Joe, this is the best picture in the whole world. Thank you God and Joe.

Monday, August 8 – Heart + 12 – Terry continues to improve. Last night I finally crashed. The adrenaline high I have had this entire time ended. I came in for a very hard landing. I was so wiped out, I got home at 6:30 in the evening and went straight to bed. I slept like a rock for almost 14 hours. After I woke up, I called the hospital to see how her night went. Her night nurse informed me she had a very restful night. They were able to not disturb her so she could get a good night sleep. Nikki and my brother and niece have gone home. Kelly went back to work and I'm on my own again. My batteries were recharged with this much needed sleep.

I called again on my way to the hospital for an update. They told me she was sitting in the chair and both the occupational and physical therapists had been there to start working with her. Both therapists would be coming in twice a day to work with Terry. The physical therapist is working with her major muscle groups. I never realized the muscles would atrophy in such a short time. She is very weak and barely able to move her arms and legs.

Dr. May came today for his daily visit, before I got there. Now that the ventilator was out, Terry asked him in a whispering voice, "Dr. May, either do this procedure or let me go home."

With a puzzled look on his face, he said, "Terry we did the transplant two weeks ago. You have a new heart and it is working wonderfully."

Later when I arrived and she told me, I realized she had no memory of anything we told her the last four days. Not the surgery, not the passage of time, not the coma. Terry developed a thrush infection in her mouth as a result of the ventilator tube being in for so long. This infection is caused by bacteria. Thrush is basically a yeast infection. What I did not know then was how hard it would be to eliminate. At this point she is very weak. For all of you who have asked about her milkshake and cinnamon bun, she has not had them. Before you all shoot me, allow me to explain. Remember they had to retrain her lungs so she could get off the ventilator. Now they have to retrain her trachea. The occupational therapist is having Terry take small sips of water and swallow them. If she starts coughing, the trachea didn't close and the water went into the lungs. From there they progress to ice chips, to see if she can shallow them . Then they move to strained foods, and finally, regular food. Trust me, she will have her treats just as soon as it's safe. Now that she is getting out of the woods, we are finding out more from the doctors about just how close she was to death that first night. Thank God for watching over her and making her one hell of a fighter.

Heart + 12 Responses:

So happy for both of you that Terry is doing better and improving day by day!

Terry is beyond TIMEX, she is SUPER WOMAN, WONDER WOMAN, BAT WOMAN, and whatever tough broad is out there combined.

Joe, Good news and it takes time. When Wes broke his leg it didn't take long for the leg muscles to atrophy and it took him several weeks before he could walk again to get most of the strength back.

Glad to hear she is moving forward. Be patient as things return to their new normal.

Yes, Thank God for keeping her here for all of us. Thank you, Joe, for taking the time to keep us informed on her recovery. Love you guys.

Unfortunately I know the situation (muscle breakdown, therapist, swallow test, etc.) all too well with my dad. Thanks for letting me know how tough the first night was. I will continue to pray for Terry's speedy recovery. She's very lucky to have such a loving and supportive husband like you and I like to see her fighting spirit! Keep it up [This writer's Dad suffered a stroke after his LVAD was installed. He has experienced a rough recovery, but like Terry, he is still fighting. Our hearts and prayers go out to them.]

Wow, it sounds really good still praying please keep me updated. Love Lisa

Tuesday, August 9 – Heart + 13 – Today was not like any other day; it will go down as *The Day of Terry's Rebellion.* Upon arriving at the ICU and buzzing for entrance, I was told I would have to wait 45 minutes before I could get in. This seemed odd to me since I knew they completed all her tests for the day, including her physical and occupational therapy.

Upon entering the unit, I was met at the door by her nurse, Susan. She proceeded to fill me in before I reached Terry's room. My hardheaded wife was sitting in the recliner. Terry decided to go to the bathroom on her own and not call for help. Her legs were not strong enough to support her. She slid down the front of the chair onto the floor. With her voice is still weak and barely above a whisper and her call button out of reach, she lay there, helpless. Fortunately she wasn't hurt.

A man walking past her room noticed her. He was afraid to enter the room so he remained in the hall, yelled for a nurse and they came running. They covered the floor with blankets and rolled her onto them. Then they rolled her on her side and washed half her body with the disinfectant soap. Then placed a fresh blanket on the floor and rolled her on to it and washed the other half of her body. The staff had to be extremely careful as she still had the staples in her chest from the surgery. The procedure was reversed and she now was completely on fresh blankets and in a new gown. It took a combination of seven nurses and technicians to safely pick her up and put her back in the chair without pulling or hurting her chest.

To prevent this from happening again, they placed a chair under the leg portion of the recliner as a wedge. This prevented her from putting the recliner in the upright position to get up. As an additional precaution they attached an alarm to the back of her gown. If she leans forward too much, the alarm trips. Later in the afternoon she asked if I would get her some fresh water. While I was at the water machine guess what went off. Yes, the alarm! She was trying to get up again, this time from the bed.

Now they not only have her gown wired, they also activated the bed's alarm system.

That evening we had our first dinner together since July 26. She had beef stroganoff with carrots and mushroom soup, Jello and iced tea. I had graham crackers and diet ginger ale. By now I'm sure you guessed what she had for dessert: her Silver Diner chocolate milkshake. I don't believe anyone has gone through so much or suffered so long to earn a chocolate milkshake. I think this could qualify for the Guinness World Records!

I stayed until 9 p.m., kissed her goodnight and said to her, "Don't give the nurses any trouble tonight!"

Her response to me was, "Don't you boss me around!" Guess my feisty little Italian is back.

Heart + 13 Responses:

Good grief she continues to make your life exciting. Hopefully she stays put long enough to heal some more.

Great news Joe, keep smiling!

Joe, please tell Terry Nora and I are thinking of her.

She sounds like she is getting antsy to get out. Keep feeding her the milkshakes.

Well it started out bad, middle good; end great, sounds like Aunt Terry is getting back to normal. Well as normal as a Geraci can be. Love and prayers Lisa

LOL, does that bring back memories! When my husband was in ICU he did the same thing. I would spend all day trying to keep him in the bed or in the chair. He even bit me one time because I put my arm across him to stop him from getting up. Good thing he was out of it when he did it or I would have decked him. When the doctors came in afterward they had that "better you than me" look on their faces. Good luck keeping her down, stay patient and give her my best.

WOW! What an improvement in just a few days. I'm so happy

for you both. Please give her a hug from me and let her know John and I can't wait to welcome her home.

This is great! How much longer do they think she will be in ICU? You are at Fairfax, right?

God bless you both for all that you have been through and continue to go through. It is times like these that really test your faith, and you realize how precious and fragile life is. I firmly believe that attitude has a lot to do with it – I saw it my Mom, and Terry is obviously a fighter as well. I'm so glad Terry is doing so well. Before you know it she'll be back out there working in the yard! Take care and God bless.

I guess she is getting back to herself again (we hope).

You're in trouble now.

I didn't know Terry was an escape artist!! No highwire until she fully healed! That was a great picture with her milkshake. Thanks for including us in the emails.

Well let's just say some things never change? She's a feisty one!

Can we assume that her alarm system goes home with her?

Wednesday, August 10 – Heart + 14 – Today was supposed to be road trip day. She was finally leaving the ICU and moving to the step down Telemetry Unit. We waited, but it did not happen. Due her continual escape attempts, they need a room next to the nurses' station so they can keep a close eye on her. While we were waiting she had a very busy day with three sessions of physical therapy. The therapist is concentrating on strengthening her legs. The best part of the day was when we all played a joke on the new technician (used to be called a nurse's aide or candy striper). She came in to help get Terry into the chair and asked about the chair alarm. When she found out what it was she said, "Oh my God, this is the patient that fell!" Then she noticed all of Terry's black and blue bruises from surgery. She was shocked, thinking how badly Terry was injured from the fall. El Vee, her nurse today, has a warped sense of humor like me and continued to play into it and build on it. We all had this poor young lady going. Even Terry joined in before we finally let her know the truth. Everybody then shared a good laugh.

Now that Terry is going to leave the ICU, I wondered if she would overcome ICU syndrome. The staff tells me they don't know what really causes it, but once the patient leaves, so does the syndrome. What is this syndrome? Basically, it's hallucinations. Terry's favorite featured the two rooms across the hall from her. One was a small nurses' lounge where they would eat lunch or go on coffee break. Next to it was a storeroom. Both doors are adjoining each other. To Terry, this was a 24-hour restaurant she wanted to try because it was busy all the time and the food was really good. She knew that, just from the delicious smell and the number of customers that were coming and going. Another hallucination was that the hospital would rent out the rooms when they had no patients. By doing this, they could keep their costs down. Whenever she started talking about these stories, we would just agree or ask questions. It surprised me how in-depth her belief in them was. For example, she told me about a family with three children who moved in next door to her. Then she started to describe the kids and their ages. The family was homeless and grateful to the hospital for the cheap rent plus all their meals were included.

While she was in the coma she had no memory of anything or even our voices. What she did remember was the recurring dreams, like the one of the devil sitting on a stepladder in the corner, telling her she was a bad girl.

Then he would chase her around the room trying to catch her. Another dream was that of people planning her funeral and another one of her mom, who kept telling her to go back, it wasn't time. From my perspective, I'm glad the devil didn't catch her. We didn't plan her funeral (though I did come close on several occasions). I'm glad her mom kept telling her to go back. I know our minds can sometimes play tricks with us and if dreams were a way for her to keep fighting to stay alive, then I'm grateful.

Heart + 14 Responses:

Sound like our aunt, sister-in-law, wife, mother, grandmother is finally coming back. Love and prayers Lisa

Sounds like Terry is getting back to normal, give her our love and hugs.

Joe it was really good seeing you this morning. I know all of this has been a bit of a nightmare for you and for Terry. Just wanted to let you know we are pulling for you both. Keeping your sense of humor the way you have is, in my opinion, the best way to survive something like this. Bless you both.

I have been following your emails about Terry's progress. Have not replied but our best wishes and prayers have always been with you Terry. That's one feisty lady but I think support has a lot to do with her recovery. Let us know if there is any way we can help. Give my best to Terry and you get some rest. We will catch up.

CHAPTER 8

Chapter 8: Step Down and Discharge

I had not sent out any updates for the last several days and people have begun to wonder if everything is okay. So today, with only a few minutes left before midnight, I emailed this update:

Saturday, August 13, 2011 – Heart + 17 – Let me begin by telling you why you have not heard from me for the last three days. Something new has been added to the equation. It's a little something called work. For some reason, those pesky bills will not take a holiday. Due to this new equation, I will be consolidating updates.

After Terry's move into the step down Telemetry Unit Wednesday night, August 10, they gave her a new blood pressure medication. She had an adverse reaction to it. Instead of lowering her blood pressure, the medication caused it to spike, and she became very nauseous. By the time her blood pressure was under control, it was dawn on Thursday, and she was exhausted. She slept for most of the day to regain her strength. Needless to say it was not a good day.

Yesterday, Friday, was good for her and bad for me. She resumed physical therapy and her legs are gradually getting stronger. Plus today, they removed the staples from her chest. I, on the other hand, have a different story to tell. As I was driving home from the hospital, my van started shooting smoke out from the vents, radio and under the dashboard. After figuring out it wasn't an electrical fire, I could see the engine was overheating. Further investigation revealed a blown heater core. No, I'm not a super mechanic; I just saw a pool of antifreeze on the passenger side of the van. By the time I got towed back to Manassas and home it was almost 11 p.m.

Today, Terry is doing much better. She can get in and out of bed by herself and into the chair. She still needs two people to assist her while she walks. Terry is still very weak and exhausts her energy very quickly. Something is going on with her digestive tract at this time. Her cardiologists brought in a gastroenterologist and he ordered a series of tests to determine what the problem is. Leading indicators are a GI infection of some type. We needed to wait for the test results to come back on Monday. Terry will also have her second heart biopsy on Monday as well. Tomorrow, Sunday, I will be working all day and not going to the hospital until Monday afternoon. It's nice that work has picked up – the extra cash inflow will come in handy. Managing finances during this ordeal hasn't been easy, but we have been holding our own. Doing a reverse mortgage on the house has been a real blessing and allowed us to use the monthly mortgage money to pay the additional medical expenses, the medicine co-pays and to slowly pay down our debt.

The transplant team ordered all of the prescription

medication Terry will require upon discharge. Once I have received them I have to bring them all to the hospital. The transplant coordinator has to verify all the drugs are on hand. She cannot be discharged until all the meds are on hand.

I have asked the staff to restrict her visitors and remove her phone from the room at this time. Currently she just doesn't have enough energy to talk, visit and rehab. As soon as she is ready, I will let you know.

Heart + 17 Responses:

Joe… I am just so thankful for your updates and for how well Terry is doing. I also love the humor you add, it is the only way to get through all of this! I am continuing to pray for both of you.

Sorry to hear about the new set of challenges you are facing. I'm hoping all will be resolved quickly.

Good morning, Joe. Please make sure you are eating well and getting rest, too. She will need you to be strong when she gets home. All my best to you, Terry and family, Warm regards.

Make sure you catch a cat nap for yourself. You have been running on super adrenaline and need to catch your breath.

Leaving town for two weeks, but will try to read emails. Don't know if you realized it but Rita is a heart transplant patient. Take care of yourself.

Wow…With everything else going on, you didn't need car trouble.

Wednesday, August 17, 2011 – Heart + 21 – Tomorrow is Terry's birthday. This will be the second straight birthday spent in the heart center; of her last five birthdays, four were in hospitals. Last birthday, she had the LVAD surgery; this year, the transplant. Other people take vacations. We just take hospitalcations.

Hopefully she'll never have to spend another birthday in the hospital. I'm planning a small birthday party for her. I have ordered birthday cake decorated with a big heart on it, plus bunch of balloons. The cake is chocolate with cream cheese icing (her favorite). She will be blown away because she is not expecting anything. Terry always claims to hate it when I surprise her, but she enjoys it. Both Kelly and I will be there, plus two of our neighbors and our friend, Susanna Barolin, to help celebrate her birthday.

All of the tests the gastroenterologist ordered for her digestive tract came back negative. The conclusion is that her digestive ailments were caused by a residual effect of the amount of anesthesia she received.

Kelly got permission today to wheel her mom out to the healing garden here at the hospital. It's in a nice secluded courtyard. It is very quiet and relaxing except when the medevac helicopter is coming in for a landing. The outdoor healing garden is a great place to read, have lunch or just relax. This was the first time in three weeks Terry was outdoors and she loved it. Even with her mask on, she could feel the warm sun on her face. Wow, what a pick-me-up for her just to venture out without carrying 16 extra pounds of equipment. They stayed outside for about an hour. Terry enjoyed the warm sun while Kelly completed some paperwork she brought from her office.

Heart + 21 Responses:

Please wish Theresa a very Happy Birthday from me... tomorrow! Please tell her that I know she is going to have a magical year. Hope all is going well.

Thursday, August 18, 2011 – Heart + 22 – Today is Terry's first REBIRTHDAY and it was very busy for her. Early in the day, two of our neighbors paid her a surprise visit. She was so happy to see someone other than family.

Later in the afternoon, I showed up with our dear friend Susanna Barolin from the City Square Café in Manassas. Of course, we brought the balloons, a chocolate cake with cream cheese icing and the birthday presents. Terry was so thankful of all the cards she received. She wanted to pass along a super thank you to Susan Jacobs for a YouTube birthday video and to all the members of my networking group, Prince William Professional Networkers, for the absolutely wonderful gift they gave her. It was a very soft, plush and warm bathrobe. She just loves it. After all that, cutting the cake was kind of anticlimactic. Confucius says, "A picture is worth a thousand words," so gaze on 5,000 words. If she continues to progress, Terry will be coming home on Monday, August 22.

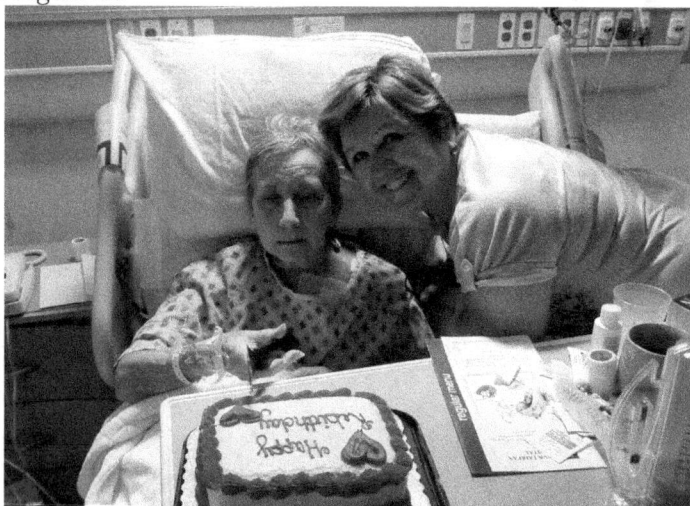

Our friend Susanna Barolin helps us celebrate Terry's Birthday.

* * *

Heart + 22 Responses:

Happy Birthday and many, many, many more! Thanks for sending such an upbeat report; it's wonderful to have good news to celebrate on Terry's birthday.

God Bless Uncle Joe Aunt Terry

Happy Birthday to Terry! Please let her know we are thinking of her!

Happy birthday Aunt Terry in all my thoughts and prayers I love, love, love, love you your niece Lisa

Joe, please wish Terry Happy Birthday for me. While it's too bad that she has to be in the hospital, there's much to celebrate.

Fantastic Joe, thank you for all the updates we'll see you when we see you.

HOME ON MONDAY? That's fantastic! Just so she behaves. John and I both wish her a very happy birthday! Hope she enjoyed her cake and ate it, too. You have been amazing through all this, Joe. I'm sure you are exhausted. It will be nice to have her home where you both can rest and relax a bit. Love you both.

Happy Birthday, Terry. Sending hugs and prayers your way.

Wish her a HAPPY BIRTHDAY for me.

Awesome about Monday! I'll keep my fingers crossed. Remember if you need anything I'm next door.

Please wish Terry a Happy Birthday!! She's in good company, my daughter's birthday was the 17th and my brother's is the 20th. That is such great news about going home. I'm praying all goes well the next few days.

Thank you so much for sending all the updates on Terry to our daughter until I had our email up and running. She forwarded them all of them to me yesterday and I had a great time reading them and seeing the pictures. Terry looks wonderful and I would love to be near so I could visit with her. I really do miss our talks on the phone and getting together now and then. Terry, your progress is remarkable; you are a living, breathing miracle. You are an inspiration to everyone and I admire you greatly. You both are in my prayers and thoughts almost daily. Keep getting better each day. I will give Terry a call when she gets home, keeping in mind not to wear her out talking. Much love and blessings.

Terry, you are one hell of a fighter and you are going to come out a winner. In fact you are already a winner in my eyes. You have certainly come a long way, baby.

Monday, August 22 – Heart + 26 – For the next five days Terry continued with her physical and occupational therapy. P/T works on building the muscles, O/T teaches simple activities like showering, the proper way to get up out of a bed and chairs, and dressing without injuring her chest.

Terry had her third heart biopsy and heart catheterization yesterday. If they went well, she could go home late in the evening today. I worked all day Saturday and Sunday in anticipation of her coming home. Once she is home she is my responsibility 24/7. We both were looking forward to it.

As luck would have it, she wasn't going home. When they did the right heart catheterization, her squeeze and output numbers were low. This could be the result of either one of two things. First, the calculations are determined by several variables; if the variables are incorrect, the output numbers are incorrect, also. Second, the heart may be showing signs of rejection. Now we will have to wait for the biopsy results to see if that's the case. If the heart is being rejected, they will treat her with higher doses of the anti-rejection drugs, Cellcept (mycophenolate mofetil) and Prograf (tacrolimus). Plus, she will spend more days in the hospital. The doctors ordered an echocardiogram for this morning to obtain additional information on the performance of the new heart.

I spent the rest of the afternoon playing cheerleader, attempting to boost Terry's spirits. She was very disappointed about not going home. In case you're wondering I didn't pull out my skirt and pompoms, it's only because they were in the trunk of the car and it was too far of a walk.

I got permission to take her outside into the healing garden again, but while the technician went for a wheelchair, the incision from the heart catheterization started bleeding. As a result, she had to remain flat in bed for the rest of the day. I stayed with Terry until about 8 p.m. and helped her eat dinner. It's kind of hard to eat when you are lying flat. We were both happy to see this day end. Tomorrow the sun will shine.

Heart + 26 Responses:

New day … New prayers … Setbacks are only temporary, although the sight of you in a skirt would cause me a setback.

Special, special prayers going up for both of you!

We'll increase the prayers. Please hang in there.

Continued support and prayers for you both and for all the organ donors you have inspired! Dr. T

Tony and I continue to lift you and Terry up in prayer. Continue to hold fast to our loving Savior for your strength and comfort! God bless and we love you both so much.

Sometimes you have to take one step back before you can take two forward. Be patient she will be home before you know it. Have a great day.

I hope everything will get better for you and Terry. I am sure she is a strong lady and she will come through this hurdle as well. My prayers and wishes are with you both.

I wish her all the best; give her a hug and a kiss for me.

Lifting you both up in prayer!

Tuesday, August 23 – Heart + 27 – I had lunch today at Panda Express in Manassas before going to the hospital. I opened the fortune cookie and it read, "Something glamorous and exciting is going to happen." Little did I know at the time that an earthquake was going to happen at 1:51 p.m. and Terry was coming home! Who says you can't believe in fortune cookies? Wish I looked closer at those six lucky numbers.

When I arrived at the hospital, I learned of the earthquake. At first, I thought they were pulling my chain. The nurses replied, "No, look at the TV!" I guess that explains why my car didn't want to go where I was steering it.

Terry's biopsy came back as a 1, with no rejection. Remember, a transplant recipient will only get a 0 if the organ is from an identical twin; if not, a 1 is great. The echocardiogram was also good, so Dr. May decided she could come home. Looks like the calculations were wrong; "garbage in, garbage out" was proven again.

Terry and I left the hospital for good, and we arrived home at 5:42 p.m. It was two hours shy of being exactly one month to the hour that we received the call about the heart becoming available. I got Terry settled in, and while she was napping, I pressed my nurse's uniform.

Heart + 27 Responses:

EXCELLENT, EXCELLENT NEWS!

YAY! Hope this means you can both get some well-deserved rest. I'm sure she will sleep better in her own bed and I know you can use some down time. Please let me know when it would be a good time to come by for a few minutes just to say hello. I don't want to be a pest. So glad she is home!

I am so glad to hear she's home and on the mend. Thank God for earthquakes. You guys must have known I was new to the area, so, you are indoctrinating me with everything: snowstorms, earthquakes and what I'm used to, hurricanes. I could live without all of it! **WELCOME HOME!**

Welcome home! I will call Terry in the near future (as I am sure your phone is ringing now more than you care to answer) please let me know if can do anything.

Hi Nurse Joe, I just got back in town from NYC and I'm catching up on my emails. First, please wish Terry a belated birthday for me. Second, I wanted to let you know I've been praying for a speedy recovery for Terry and I'm so happy she is back home although this morning I woke up realizing that since my dad had a clinic appointment I could swing by and give her a big hug and kiss. I was going to ask Tonya if that would be okay. Now you will have to give the hug and kiss for me. Tell her I love her, too, and I'm so happy for her and you and your entire family. Be well – talk soon.

Such wonderful news! What a blessing to have your precious wife home again. Thank you, Lord for your hand upon T&J and bringing the work that was done on the operating table to completion with healing. It is in you that we live, and move, and have our being. We only breathe because you let us. And may the spiritual work that was begun in their hearts continue to grow so that with each day they will be closer to you, and may they know that Jesus Christ is Lord, to the glory of God. Amen.

Thanks for the continued updates, Joe. Glad she is at home. I'm sure you both will be more comfortable.

Great news Uncle Joe! I would just love to see your legs in that nurse's dress.

I'm so happy for you both. Fabulous! Way to go Joe & Terry

Fabulous! WOOHOOO!

This is fantastic news! I'm so happy to hear you're home! I went and gave platelets for you today. I'm making something for you and when I finish, I hope you'll feel up to a visit. Take good care of her Joe, nursing is a tough job.

Terry going home is great news – Praise God! We continue to keep you all in our thoughts and prayers as you both walk the road of recovery! We love and miss you guys. Hoping to take a trip back east to visit! God Bless!

Great news J&T! Welcome back home, now comes the test to see how good a nurse you will be. Lots of Love!

Awesome, when will she be able to have visitors?

Well I guess you will remember the day you came home as well as the day you received the call. I'm going to assume everything was fine in and out of the house. Robert and I were driving on I-66 and did not feel a thing when the earthquake hit. I'm not going to call you because you are the nurse. So I will be checking emails. Give Terry our love, and let me know if we can be of any help. We are here for you.

Joe, I'm so glad to hear the good news! Congrats to you and Terry.

Uncle Joe, since you won't turn into a lady you might as well get your skirt pressed. Take lots of pictures all my love, love your niece Lisa.

Here's a really big welcome home, Terry. I'm sure you are happy to be home and in your own bed and around your own things. They really took great care of you at the heart center. Kudos to all the doctors, staff and Joe! Joe truly was your rock. Way to go, Joe. Terry you fought so hard and it really did pay off – big time. We are praising God! Thanks for emails and continue to improve. We love you and think of you each day.

So what's your whistle song while you iron your nurse uniform? Reply: Kiss my A--! Sorry I don't know that one, how does it go?

CHAPTER 9

Chapter 9: Recovery at Home

While my daily "Heart +" emails ended, I continued to send out a summary email every week or two to family and friends. Some of their responses are included here.

Our first week home has just flown by. Both of us are still adjusting to all the transplant protocols. Terry can't go out in public for another two months and is housebound (I call it house arrest, but she hates when I say that). She is still "transplant hot." When she leaves the house she has to wear a mask. She can't dig or do any kind of gardening until next summer. All foods have to be washed before she can eat them. This includes even the peels of oranges and melons. If you do not wash the exterior, what's on the outside will be transferred by the knife to the inside of the fruit. She can't ever eat at a buffet or salad bar. Nor can she ever have a grapefruit or anything with grapefruit in it. No alcohol for one year, and then, only a glass of wine, sparingly. Both grapefruit products and alcohol affect the levels of the anti-rejection drug in her blood and could cause rejection.

These are all precautions needed because her immune system has been suppressed. Anyone coming into the house for the next three months has to wash and disinfect their hands, plus Terry will have to wear a mask while they are here and sit at the opposite side of the room. At work, if I do demolition or other dusty jobs, I will have to strip down in the garage and bag up my clothes before going into the house. I have to place the contaminated clothes in the washer so the risk of infection is minimized. Then I must shower before getting near her. Germs and molds that are harmless to you and me could be fatal to her.

Today, Tuesday, August 30, 2011, she had her clinic appointment and heart biopsy. We will know the results of the biopsy tomorrow. If the results remain at 1, the level of anti-rejection drugs will be lowered again. We are still searching for the balance between rejection and maximizing her immune system. She was able to walk from the parking garage into the hospital for her appointments and back to car with the help of a walker. Once we returned home, she was exhausted and spent the afternoon napping. Terry started her in home physical therapy last Friday. The therapist will be coming three times a week for six weeks.

On top of everything else she is dealing with, now we have a new problem. Because the Foley catheter was in for almost a month she now is experiencing problems with her bladder. The medical staff at the hospital figured it would remedy itself. Again, she couldn't be that lucky. The problem was her bladder kept sending out signals every few minutes that she needed to urinate. These were false alarms about 95 percent of the time.

So now she needed to see a urologist. I found one in the

area who was in our insurance network and made an appointment for her. One more doctor on the contact list. I took her to the first appointment and the doctor examined her and told her she was suffering from an overactive bladder. This was a common problem, especially if one has been on a Foley catheter for any extended time. The urologist prescribed a medication for her and wanted to see her back in three weeks. Three weeks later, she was back. The first medication had done absolutely nothing to resolve the problem. So her doctor prescribed another medication. If this one didn't work, the doctor suggested the next step would be a 12-week procedure done in her office. Fortunately this new prescription worked. I could tell Terry really did not want to have 12 weeks of additional appointments.

Responses:

Great news Joe. Hope her progress continues.

Great report. You will soon be trying to keep up with her. Please give her my best and tell her I am thinking of her. I'm hoping to see her at one of our future shows.

I'm so glad you know where to find me if you want to talk.

Thank you so much for keeping us up-to-date on Terry's progress. She is always on our minds and in our prayers. We ordered a welcome home plant for her. I'm hoping she received it okay.

Just to let you know, I really miss the updates on Terry. They were so great to hear how she was improving daily. I especially miss your witty comments. You missed your calling, kid; you should have been a writer. Love to Terry. Please tell her we are all pulling for her. Oh be sure you keep up on your duties as chief cook and bottle washer. I'm sure your dinners are greatly enjoyed by Terry. Love you both!

Today is Tuesday, September 13, and marks Terry's third week at home. As the caregiver and well spouse, I find that there are just not enough hours in the day. Progress is slow but she continues to move forward. Of course, if you ask her, she can't figure out why she is not running a marathon.

Terry is still housebound and beginning to suffer from cabin fever. Since the weather is still nice she sits out on the deck or on the front porch. Olivia has let Granny have Buddy for a couple of weeks again. So wherever she goes, Buddy goes. He is her little shadow. She loves having him around to keep her company. Buddy loves it because of the constant attention he's getting. I have started looking in earnest for a small dog for her. I have visited the local animal shelters and left my information so I could be notified when one becomes available.

Her biopsy last week was good and her rejection drug levels were lowered again. They started reducing the level of steroids she has been taking. The steroids give her the shakes. Terry is still battling the thrush infection in her mouth. They have now changed her meds for this to what is called Miracle mouthwash. You have to go to one of the old-fashioned drugstores where they still mix the drugs. Hopefully this will knock it out. The problem is her immune system. With it being so suppressed, it's not easy to fight even simple infections. The physical therapist, Linda, works her pretty good. Terry can now go up and down the stairs on her own and she walks up and down the driveway several times a day. Personally I think it's great that someone else is telling her what to do instead of me. She is now able to take care of herself during the day while I get some work done. I'm still fighting those pesky bills.

I get everything ready and laid out for her before I leave. In the evening when I get home I get dinner ready and get whatever else done that I need to do in the evening. Her two-month anniversary is fast approaching. It is really hard to believe she only has one more month on house arrest.

Terry is now getting very antsy and suffering from a bad case of cabin fever. She really looks forward to her clinic visits. They are an opportunity for her to get out and interact with other people. She had a visit from her former coworker Phyllis last week. Phyllis retired and moved to South Carolina. She was back in the area for a wedding and came by to visit Terry. They spent the afternoon together catching up. The visit did wonders for Terry's morale.

Terry has made tremendous progress this past week. Even she can see the improvements she is making. I like to believe it is because I read her the riot act a couple of weeks ago. She did not want to do her breathing exercises, nor eat because of her sore mouth. The medication still is not working to clear up her mouth infection and now she is on another drug that is even stronger. She has to get added blood work as a result because this new drug causes the anti-rejection drug levels to fluctuate in her body. Basically I told her not to come crying to me.

"If you want to get better, you need to eat even if your mouth hurts," I told her. "You can't run a car with no gas in the tank. If you want your breathing to improve then you need to do the breathing exercises. I know it is uncomfortable and it hurts. You didn't cut me any slack when I had to do them after my knee surgery so you're not going to get any sympathy from me."

I think I finally got through to my stubborn little Italian. Yesterday she had a physical therapy evaluation and did okay. She has begun to walk around the cul-de-sac twice a day, plus she goes up and down the stairs several times a day. She has taken over doing her own morning and evening medical procedures and now fixes her own lunch. All of this has lightened my load. Last night for the first time she started reading her first book since the transplant. I am so proud of her. Her weekly heart biopsy was good again this week and the level of anti-rejection drugs was lowered again. Hopefully next week she will be off the steroids completely and perhaps the shaking will stop. This next week we will have Monday, Tuesday and Wednesday full of doctor's appointments either for me or for her. You know you are getting old when everyone in your contact list of names begins with "Doctor."

Responses:

Thanks for sending the update. So glad to hear Terry is progressing so well and they've been able to lower her anti-rejection drugs. That's definitely a good sign plus her increased stamina building. Hang in there Mr. Mom!

Tell her to keep up the good work and God will do the rest.

Thanks for the update sounds like everything is going as planned, slow and steady.

Good for pushing the P/T and eating. There was a lot of P/T when my mom had a stroke and it's crucial. This is the only treatment with no side effects or risk. Sometimes it really seems like it takes "determination" to get the best results, not just cooperation. Sounds like you gave her determination.

I'm so glad to hear about Terry's progress. I am sure she is getting stronger each day. You are a godsend to her and a wonderful husband

and there are not many of you around. I know as I have a husband like you who is very helpful in a time of need. Terry is a lucky girl, and I am sure the two of you will continue to grow old together gracefully and without any further episodes of ill health. It is the Jewish New Year starting on Wednesday and you are in my prayers.

This really wonderful news that Terry is making tremendous progress is very exciting! I'm so happy for your family & will continue to keep your family in my thoughts and prayers. I left a voicemail on her cell last week and noticed the recording was in your voice. When will she be able to be on her cell taking calls again? I'm looking forward to seeing all of you soon. xoxoxo

[Here is an email exchange I had with my niece who has a doctorate. The two of us always try to yank each other's chain. She takes after her dad, my late brother, Sal.]

So happy to see al the progress!

Me: For you Doctorates the correct spelling is "all" and not al

Uncle Smart A--! Shouldn't you be cooking or cleaning or some other important thing.…..? And not worrying about my spelling.

Whenever someone calls or visits Terry, they always ask if she has seen or read the email updates I was doing. I saved them for her until she would be able to read them. Finally today she asked if I would print them out. I printed about a 150 pages before I remembered I could just copy and paste. I put them in a binder for her. As she was reading them she started to cry. I asked her, "Why are crying?"

Her reply was, "You made out to be a hero and I'm no hero."

I said, "Yes, you are. Your fight and your strength and determination have moved inspired and uplifted people. Because of you, people have given blood and platelets and

158

made the decision to be organ donors. You are definitely a hero in my book."

We moved into October 2011 and the news continues to be bright. The heart catheterization and biopsy were good and she is now officially off house arrest and off the steroids completely. To celebrate, tonight we went out to dinner. Next week the doctors will complete the paperwork for the Division of Motor Vehicles so her driver's license can be reinstated and she will be able to drive again. Life is beginning to take on some normalcy around here. It's been so long, I don't know if I will be able to handle it. Come December, I'm scheduled to have other knee replaced and come next spring we both should be able to PARTY!

October also means my arts & crafts show season starts in earnest. This year I had a number of shows out of town. Two of the five weekends in October, I was on the road. While I was gone, our daughter, Kelly kept looking in on her mom. We finished the weekly heart biopsies and are getting them done monthly. So far each has been rated a 1 and the anti-rejection drug levels keep getting reduced. Terry has lost about 10 pounds since the surgery. Her mouth still has the thrush infection. She is trying a third different medicine now and it is having some improvement. Of course, she's been there before. Every time we think it's on the run, it flares back with a vengeance. One Thursday morning she came with me to my Prince William Professional Networkers meeting to personally thank them for the birthday present and all of their kind wishes and prayers.

In November I have two shows up north, one in

western New York and the other in Western Pennsylvania. I like doing these shows because I can visit with the family in Buffalo and my daughter Nikki and her husband, Sean, in Erie. We cleared with the medical staff and this year Terry could come with me. While I worked the shows she would visit with my sisters-in-law and our daughter. On Sunday while my brother Augie and I worked the show, Terry went to lunch with both my sisters-in-law, all the nieces and grandnieces. She really had fun and enjoyed herself. I loved having her with me on the road again. Even though she wasn't involved with the shows, it was nice just to travel and be together again. She had a wonderful time; it was nice to see that old smile again. When she was tired she would take a nap. One evening after dinner while we were at our daughter Nikki's home our son-in-law, Sean, started looking for dogs up for adoption on the Internet. He found several. Some were at the local chapter of the ASPCA (American Society for the Prevention of Cruelty to Animals) in Erie; the others were at an animal shelter just over the state line in Ohio. So we decided the next day would be spent looking for a pet. Since the ASPCA in Erie was closer, we started there. They had a lot of Huskies and I thought for sure Nikki and Sean would bring home one of them. You see, they had already adopted four of them. They are, as we say, our "granddogs." I keep teasing Nikki and Sean by saying, "You need two more, then at least you'd have a dog sled team."

As for the small dogs, there weren't many from which to choose. Most were Chihuahuas except for one little guy named Poochie who was a Pomeranian mix. He looked so scared in that cage, but I really liked him. He was cute and had personality. Terry just sort of blew by him and started looking at other dogs. She liked one named Sally who was a Beagle mix. We then met with the attendant who brought Sally into the get-acquainted room. Sally was very active and weighted about 35 to 40 pounds. Sally the Beagle thought she was lap dog and liked the attendant more than us. Even though she was cute and Terry really liked her, she would be too much dog for Terry to handle.

I suggested Poochie, the Pomeranian mix. Terry wasn't too enthused, but agreed to get acquainted. As soon as Poochie came into the room and was off the lead he jumped right into her lap and started licking her face. That was all it took. Terry fell in love with him and he was coming home with us. Terry didn't know it at the time, but before we went into the room I went back and had a talk with Poochie. I told him, "Now, be sure to go to Terry first and jump in her lap. If you will do that, Poochie, you will have a home." I know it sounds funny, but it was a trick I learned years earlier.

You see, right after Nikki got out of grad school she was working in State College, Pennsylvania. I stopped in to visit with her on my way back from Buffalo. She and her roommate had this kitten named Madison. Their landlord found out about the kitten and he would not allow a pet in the apartment, so they had to get rid of Madison. So Nikki asked me to take Madison home with me, just like she had done with our other cat, "Miss Kitty." Now Miss Kitty was your typical independent leave-me-alone cat who did not like to be petted or held. Terry said the next cat we get, had to be the opposite or we could not have it. So on the way home I told Madison what she needed to do if she wanted a home. As I walked in the door I knew

Terry was not happy that I had brought home another cat. But when I let Madison out of the travel cage, she jumped into Terry's lap and settled in for the duration. After that "Maddie" found a home.

We completed all the paperwork and sure enough, Poochie left with us. On the way to the car, Terry renamed him "Eddie" and for the rest of time at Nikki and Sean's house they were inseparable. Eddie sat on her lap the entire drive home. Eddie looks like "Toto" from *The Wizard of OZ*, only he's black and not charcoal gray. At night at our daughter's home, he slept between us. Now he sleeps at Terry's feet at night. While she lies on the couch, he's right there next to her. Other times he gets carried, just like a baby. Please don't think he's spoiled or anything like that, but I will say, he gives the term lap dog a whole new meaning.

We got home on November 15. The following Monday, Terry had her heart biopsy and again the result was another 1. After the biopsy we had to go to another lab for a special test. It had to be another lab and not the hospital because of the Federal government. The hospital cannot even draw the blood and forward it to the other lab. So Terry had to be the pin cushion just to keep the clowns in Washington happy. What happens after they receive the results of this blood test is, they compare these test results with her heart biopsy results. This determines a baseline for her. Then, in the future, she will have the blood test once a month and the heart biopsy every third month. Plus, based on the numbers from the blood work, the doctor will also be able to adjust her levels of the anti-rejection drugs. This blood test is called Allomap®, the only non-invasive gene expression test that helps doctors identify the absence of heart transplant rejection.

She started another stronger medication for her mouth infection. Hopefully this and the new lower level of ant-rejection drugs will help overcome this mouth problem and she will be eating again. In case you are wondering, Eddie came with us and waited in the car while we were in the hospital. Sometimes we call him "Eddie L. Barker" (L is for licker, he licks you constantly; The Barker because he barks at very noise.

The only downside she experienced was that her mouth infection continues to worsen, even with the new medication. The doctor ran a test last week when she had the heart biopsy and we got the results. They discovered she not only had the bacterial infection or thrush, she also has a viral infection as well. So they added another medication to get rid of that one. As we approached Thanksgiving her appetite dropped off tremendously. Let me rephrase that: she still had the appetite; it's just her mouth hurt so bad when she ate, that she wouldn't eat. Thanksgiving added a new surprise. Now, on top of the two infections, the burning mouth syndrome was back with the painful sensations she had after chemotherapy. Now, even her teeth and gums were hurting as she chewed. This was a new element thrown into the equation.

Thanksgiving marks a new milestone for us: 120 days post-transplant. At Thanksgiving dinner we all were extremely thankful to have her with us and for her to have the gift of a new heart. The day was dampened, however, because she ate like a bird. Her mouth was really bothering her. Over the next several weeks her weight continued to drop. She would lose two to three pounds a week – some weeks, more.

Responses:

Good luck and have a blessed Thanksgiving!

I know you have plenty of family but if you or your bride need anything. I hope you know you can call to assist XXX OOO

Thank you for such a wonderful update. It warms my heart to hear my ol' Joe full of feist and spunk. I will continue to lift you and Terry and thank my God continually for his faithfulness.

Yes, government sucks, it's another reason why so many are for less of it. I'm glad she is getting better. I can picture this dog and I suspect you will find lots of joy with him as I have with mine.

It's OK for a big guy to talk to a dog, just watch who you do it in front of.

I'm so happy for the both of you. I hope her mouth gets resolved soon. Your recent trip sounds like a great success and a new dog to boot! Enjoy and savor your Thanksgiving.

Great news for the most part also a really great photo of you in the paper last week! Good Luck and have a blessed Thanksgiving. [*The Manassas Observer* published a photo of me standing by my show display on the front page of their newspaper. The caption announced I was a featured artist at an upcoming arts & crafts show.]

Congratulations on the new addition. I have four dogs and they are the joy of my life. They are with me all day when not with clients. They will give you unconditional love.

Thank you for sharing the news. I miss seeing you but think of you all the time. I've been busy with Mom the past couple of months. We hope you all have the best Thanksgiving ever.

Congrats on the new addition to the family. Pets do wonderful things to lift the spirits and promote a good immune system.

Best wishes for a happy Thanksgiving. You have so much to be thankful for this year. Blessings.

My show season ended the first weekend in December 2011 and the following week I went in to the hospital to have my other knee replaced. Before I went in, I made sure all Terry's meds were laid out for the next week. The surgery was done on December 12. Due to some minor complications, I had to stay in the hospital an additional day. Terry visited me each afternoon in the hospital and each day she appeared to be exhausted. I asked if she was eating and she would say, "Yes." I didn't know at this point that her idea of eating was just a bowl of cereal or a yogurt cup each day.

I came home on Thursday and my brother Augie and my niece came down to help out again on Friday. I was happy for that mainly because it took a load off Terry. They stayed for a week which was long enough me to be up and around at least with the help of a walker. Terry's weight continued to drop. She's down to 110 pounds and I'm getting really worried. I spoke to the transplant coordinator, Mary Beth Maydosz, about this. I wanted to know how long before they did something. In other words, did they have a "Plan B"? She said yes, they did, but wanted to wait until after the holidays. They raised the level of medication to treat her mouth and reduced the anti-rejection drugs. In fact, they eliminated the Cellcept completely to keep the necessary levels in her blood stream from spiking too high. The mouth medications would increase the anti-rejection levels to an unsafe point. All of this had to be continuously monitored for her safety.

I took Terry to her December clinic appointment. Her mouth was no better and they were afraid the infections had spread down her esophagus. Now we needed to see a gastroenterologist to have an endoscopic test done to see if the infections had indeed spread. The test was done on December 17, as an outpatient. The good news was, the infections had not spread down the esophagus.

Terry's depression was deepening at this point. She began complaining, "I've done all this and I'm no better," or "I'm worse now than before – when are they ever going to tell me the truth?" I tried to motivate her and to always be positive but it was getting very hard. Even I was becoming a Doubting Thomas. After all, we had been on this journey almost five years, and the light at the end of the tunnel keeps getting moved back. Were we ever going to have a normal life again?

We spent Christmas Eve 2011 at Kelly's house with her and Olivia. The plan was to spend the night and stay Christmas Day for dinner. After opening presents and having breakfast Christmas morning Terry and I were both exhausted. We decided not to stay for dinner. In the early afternoon we went home. Once home we both just went to bed and slept on through to the next morning. For the next week, we just muddled through. On Friday, December 31, Mary Beth called me and informed me they needed blood work done to make sure her numbers were still good. I told her I would bring Terry in first thing Monday morning.

On Tuesday, I received a call from the transplant clinic. The doctor had received the results from the blood work and the results were not favorable. We needed to be at the clinic at 9 a.m. on Wednesday, January 4, 2012. The New Year was not starting out well. I wondered just how bad things really were. The medical staff member did not give many details over the phone. The tone of voice was enough to make me worry.

CHAPTER 10

Chapter 10: Relapse

At the clinic appointment the lab technician drew more blood and then Mary Beth Maydosz examined Terry. On July 26, 2011, when she arrived at the hospital for the transplant, she weighed 136 pounds. She had lost 36 pounds in four months, 16 of those pounds in the four weeks since Thanksgiving. At this point, Terry weighed exactly 100 pounds fully clothed with shoes.

She was just skin and bones. I mean that literally. She had absolutely no meat on her. Her skin was dry, badly wrinkled and just hung there. The blood test revealed her bone marrow had stopped producing blood cells. Her kidneys were failing and she was severely dehydrated. Mary Beth calculated her approximate caloric daily intake. It amounted to less than 500 calories a day.

She then asked Terry point blank, "Can you promise me you will go home, hold your nose and drink four or five bottles of a high protein drink a day?"

When Terry replied, "No," Mary Beth's next words were, "You are going to be admitted."

I was so happy to hear Mary Beth say that. I was exhausted from arguing with Terry and forcing her to try to eat something…anything…just, please, eat. I knew it was painful but Terry just would not eat through the pain. Mary Beth put it in stark contrast for Terry: "You know those TV commercials that ask viewers to help starving children? Well, those children are in better condition than you are."

I called Kelly and Nikki and told them about their mom. Kelly would come over to the hospital after work. Terry and I sat in the hospital waiting room all day until a room became available at 5 p.m. The nurses got Terry settled into the room a few minutes later they hooked her up to an IV and started pumping in fluids to rehydrate her. Later that evening a feeding tube was inserted through her nose to start feeding her directly into her stomach. This was an immediate solution until she could have a PEG tube inserted into her stomach. A PEG tube is a percutaneous endoscopic gastrostomy tube inserted into the stomach to feed her directly. It's normally a long-term solution for someone who cannot eat orally. Now that she was taken care of, I limped off home. It had only been three weeks since my knee surgery.

Over the weekend, the hospital staff kept feeding her through a tube inserted through her nose. The transplant team brought in an infectious disease doctor, an ear, nose and throat specialist, a gastroenterologist, a nutritionist and a psychiatrist. Everyone was bringing their talents together to get her back on her feet. Monday morning they took her down for the insertion of the PEG tube. With this in place, the feeding tube was removed from her nose. That little gesture lifted her spirits. She felt embarrassed with that tube coming out of her nose. With her in the hospital, they could have constant readings of the medication levels in her system. With this information her meds could be regulated to obtain the maximum balance and healing. While this is a layman's interpretation of what they were doing, the point is, it worked, and her mouth began to finally heal. Terry spent a total of 11 days in the hospital. Over this period she gained six pounds. The medication for her mouth finally started to take effect. The left side of her mouth healed first. She could now chew and drink on the left side and was able to eat with minimum pain. During the day she would eat as much of regular foods as she could. At night she would receive the high protein feeding via the PEG tube. The nursing staff and the dietician kept track of the total amount of all the foods and fluids she consumed. For the burning mouth syndrome she was receiving B-complex vitamins and doses of zinc oxide. This, plus being hydrated and receiving high protein nourishment, was bringing Terry back to health. Her body now had the fuel to heal and fight back.

While Terry was in the hospital she started counseling with the psychiatrist. Treating the physical aspect was one thing. Now it was time to treat the mental and emotional aspects of her medical condition. Terry has been depressed for what now seemed like forever. The depression started with the breast cancer and she never really had a chance to deal with it. She just sort of controlled it by keeping it just under the surface. Now, after almost five years of ill health and no real quality of life, her mental state from battling the physical and mental trauma was taking its toll on her and keeping her from getting better. Think about it: for almost five years she did everything the medical staff asked and she was still trying to regain her health. In fact, Terry went from bad to worse. I'm a pretty positive person and even I was beginning to wonder. The psychiatrist put it this way for Terry: "You are in a deep hole. Now, it's time to stop digging, pull yourself out and fill in the hole." She started counseling sessions with the psychiatrist while she was still in the hospital, plus the psychiatrist prescribed three different anti-depression drugs to help. Currently Terry is on two, and both of those are the minimum dosages.

Responses:

I was not able to make the meeting this morning, but I wanted to wish both you and Terry a very speedy recovery.

Joe, I'm so sorry to hear about Terry's setback and your knee. You both are in my thoughts and prayers.

Dear Joe, I'm so sorry to hear about Terry. I hope you continue to keep us posted. I'm adding an extra prayer every night before I go to sleep that they soon find a reason for the mouth problems. She can't afford to lose 36 lbs. she doesn't weight that much to start with. I know God will hear them. You will also get better with your knee just keep up your P/T. Do not be dumb like me. Mine are finally starting to allow me to walk without too much pain.

Glad to hear Terry is in the hospital being taken care of. She was probably becoming malnourished. Please, if there is anything you need me to do just call. Hope she's better soon.

Give her a big hug for me!

Holy smokes, Joe. Please just let me know if there is anything I can do to help.

My best wishes are with you and Terry. Please both of you get well quick!

So saddened and surprised to hear about Terry — will keep her in my thoughts and prayers. I was going to call you about your next knee surgery for some reason I had it in my mind it was this month – will be praying for you also. If you need anything don't hesitate to ask.

I spoke to Terry before you all went away to try and coordinate seeing you both. Things have been hectic for me with Dad, work, holidays, etc. I am so sorry to hear about Terry being in the hospital. She is in my prayers. Please let me know when she is up for having visitors and I will come visit. Hang in there wishing you all the best. God Bless!

Please give Terry my best. She is in my thoughts and prayers. Eddie must be missing her. Take care of your knee. Warm Regards.

While Terry was in the hospital, Eddie was not a happy camper. Each day when I got home, I found his piles of unhappiness. He definitely does not like her not being around and not being able to see her. No matter what I did or how much I pampered him, he wanted his Mommy back.

Upon returning home, the in-line feedings would continue. The nurses at the hospital showed me how to hook up and clean the PEG tube: One more skill added to my quiver of caregiver arrows. On the day of her discharge, the hospital had coordinated with our insurance company and the insurance's medical supply vendor. The supply company delivered everything to the house: the Kangaroo feeding pump, the IV pole, the IV bags, and cans of liquid nourishment. The delivering technician showed me how to operate and load their model pump. The next day six cases of canned nourishment showed up at our doorstep. So every night for the next two weeks I fed her 1000 milliliters of the high protein nutrient spread out over 12 hours. This way she would eat as much regular food during the day as she could and while she slept she would be nourished via the PEG tube. The Kangaroo feeding pump mounted on the IV pole regulated the flow. I would set the amount to be delivered and the delivery time and the pump did the work. When her weight reached 116 pounds, we were told to stop the feedings. Her mouth continued to improve. The healed portion of her mouth kept spreading more and more to the right side her mouth. As her mouth improved so did her appetite. As of this writing (March 4, 2012) Terry has regained 25 pounds. Her skin is soft and supple. Her energy level is vastly improved and she is reading like crazy again. I'm getting my BCT back (Before Cancer Terry).

For the balance of January 2012, we remained busy with various medical appointments. I finished the physical therapy appointments for my knee and the follow-up appointment with the orthopedist. Terry had her blood drawn and her six-month heart biopsy. At her six-month clinic appointment, Mary Beth told Terry her numbers were the best they have ever been. We are beginning to feel like we could actually take a real vacation this summer – not another hospitalcation like the past two years with her LVAD surgery (2010) and heart transplant (2011).

February 2012 was another busy month. I have healed enough to start gearing up my handy man services company, plus I started writing this book. Our Valentine's Day this year was reminiscent of those long ago. Terry's PEG tube was finally removed. She gets so excited whenever she doesn't have anything hanging from her body. I tease her now she's the woman with three navels: the normal one (center), the one from the LVAD driveline (right) and the one from the PEG tube (left). February 27 was her seven-month anniversary. We celebrated by her having the monthly heart biopsy. This time, not only were the results good, she was wide awake and having lunch when I walked into recovery (previously, she would have been still knocked out for an hour to an hour and a half after the procedure). This time she was wide awake and having lunch. What a sight! Man, was I so excited! Remember when our babies were newborns, how excited we would get over their pooped diapers? Now, you got it. Normal was beautiful.

* * *

The months just keep flying by and it's already March 14, 2012. The weather is absolutely glorious outside. Terry and I are sitting on the deck. She's reading on her Barnes & Noble NOOK® and I'm writing this book on my laptop. I can't tell you just how many people encouraged me to write this book of our journey. It has definitely been that – one I never wish to duplicate, but I know how much it helped Terry and I like to hear what others before us had been through. Maybe by sharing our experiences, we might help someone in the future. Besides, getting it all down has helped me to process what I went through as the well spouse, the Nurse Joe, the Mr. Mom and the chief cook and bottle washer. What I noticed during this entire odyssey was the extremely limited amount of information available for people such as myself who have been thrust into this situation or a similar one. Hopefully they could find something here in the book to help them be better prepared, to get them thinking about what questions to ask, or even if reading this book helps them keep their sanity. If it wasn't for faith, humor and support of family, friends and strangers, I don't know if I would have survived.

Earlier this morning we both were outside working in the flower beds. Terry was so happy to be out there and gardening again. She wore her mask and gloves and was only able to work for one hour, but she was just so happy. Last week Terry had her first stress test and passed with flying colors. Dr. May was most impressed. This was the first time he saw her personally since her January 2012 hospital stay. Her weight is now up to 127 lbs. To sum it up, she is doing FANTASTIC!

Terry told Dr. May I was writing about our experiences, and when he came back through the lobby he said to me, "I hear you're writing a book, Joe. In the movie, I want George Clooney to play me."

I replied, "Dr. May, that's going to be difficult. He has more hair than you. We both laughed.

The stress test was needed to develop her heart rehab program. Hopefully next month she will start the rehab. This is very important because the heart is not connected to any nerves. The nerves to the heart are severed upon transplant. As a consequence of this, as she begins to exert herself, it takes a while for the heart to speed up and pump more. Rehab helps in this process. Think of it as another training exercise.

Responses:

I'm glad everything worked out great.

What marvelous news. She's really is a "trooper." Give her my best and congratulations. I am looking forward to seeing her at one of her upcoming shows.

Great news, Joe.

How exciting about Terry and the book. I can't wait to come to your book signing.

Joe, that's wonderful. Thank you for sharing and I'm looking forward to reading your book.

Fantastic news! So glad Terry is doing so well and glad you are writing! Thanks for the update.

That's great news about Terry. I really feel good when I hear someone recovering so well from such a major ordeal. My wife's principal wrote a book and I'm going to find out the contact for you. Will let you know as soon as I can.

Please tell Terry I said hello and send my best. I have a great book that she needs to read: The Best of Me by Nicholas Sparks. I guarantee she will enjoy it. I look forward to reading your published book, too!

Glad to hear Terry is doing fantastic!

I want one!

I'm glad everything is working out great.

Wonderful news, Joe. Please let the Squirt know we are thinking of her.

So wonderful to hear about all this.

Wow, I find it hard to believe that I have brought you up-to-date from the beginning right up to the present. I have finished going all through my journals, notes and emails to reach this point. From this point on the balance of the book will be written as events happen. You will know the ending almost the same time we do. My intent is to end the book on her first anniversary of her heart transplant, July 27, 2012.

Today, March 27, marked another milestone – her eight-month anniversary with the new heart. Yesterday she had her monthly biopsy and the results were great. The medical staff at the clinic tells her every time they listen to her heart and lungs she sounds so boring. Terry mentioned to Mary Beth, the transplant nurse practitioner that she was out gardening again. Upon hearing this Mary Beth said, "What? You can't do that until the fall. You need to wait a year."

Now it was my turn to say, "I told you so."

Terry said, "The manual says six months."

To which Mary Beth replied, "I know, and that is a misprint in the Post Heart Transplant Patient Education Manual that is being corrected."

This reminded me of what Mark Twain once said: "Be careful about reading health books. You may die of a misprint."

Now that the heart center has the results of two heart biopsies and two heart catheterizations, tomorrow I have to take her to a special lab for them to draw blood so they can do the AlloMap® test again. [Remember, the AlloMap® is the only non-invasive gene expression test that helps doctors identify the absence of heart transplant rejection]. If all works well, she will need the heart biopsy/catheterizations once every quarter and the AlloMap® the other two months. Drawing blood is a lot easier than a surgical procedure and a whole lot quicker.

The blood test results from the heart center clinic revealed her bone marrow was not producing white blood cells. Her white count was dangerously low. Remember her immune system is already comprised because of the anti-rejection drugs she is taking. The clinic called and we needed to get in there as soon as possible for a booster shot to jump start her bone marrow. Mary Beth informed Terry she would have to restrict her activities. No going out in public. Outside of our house, she would need to wear a mask even in the car if the air is not re-circulated.

Terry wanted to visit a neighbor's son who was in the hospital, but Mary Beth put a stop to that. "Hospitals have sick people and you do not need to be there any longer than necessary," she explained. So for the next week and a half we just pretty much laid low and stayed home, except for church.

***

Easter morning arrived and we attended the early Mass. Afterwards I drove her to Kelly's house. Terry was going to drive to North Carolina with Kelly to pick up Olivia. They spent the night and returned Easter Monday. Upon her return, I informed her Mary Beth had emailed me. We needed to go and have blood drawn the next day, Tuesday. They needed to check her white blood cell count, plus all the other routine things they check. Later in the afternoon she had her monthly appointment with her psychiatrist who continues to work with her on her depression.

***

We received a call today from the clinic; they had the results of yesterday's blood work. Her white blood cell count was okay, but now we had a new problem. The blood pressure medication she was taking spiked her potassium to a dangerously high level and it needed to be lowered as soon as possible. The plan was for Terry to take 20mg of Lasik (a diuretic medication) for two days and drink as much water as she could handle. On Friday, we need to have blood drawn again to check the potassium level and see if it is within the normal range again.

***

Today being Friday, we had to go have her blood drawn this morning. However; early this morning I called the clinic because Terry was very light headed, dizzy, was suffering a bad headache and plus she has a cold. This is her first cold in three years. I wanted to check if there was any over-the-counter medication she couldn't take because of all the other drugs she's taking. We do not need any other complications. The light headedness and dizziness was caused by the new blood pressure medication, so we stopped it for 24 hours. Tomorrow we will restart it and lower the dosage. Sometimes I feel like a Pharmacist because I monitor all her medications, stock her weekly pill box and order refills whenever needed.

* * *

This past Sunday, April 15, we did something we have not been able to do in almost two years. That is to have Sunday breakfast outdoors at Robert and Susanna Barolin's City Square Café. We took Eddie L. Barker with us because they allow dogs in the outside eating area. The weather was absolutely perfect. It was sunny and warm with no humidity and just a very light breeze. Mister Barker was on his best behavior and his order of bacon was cooked to perfection.

It's amazing how the older you get, the more you appreciate the little things in life. When you get right down to it, I've always said, "If you wake up in the morning, you have one more chance to make good or screw things up. The trick is waking up." I am so grateful to have this time with Terry each day. To me it is remarkable having come so close to losing her on numerous occasions as we both travelled through this odyssey. For the first time in a very long time our lives are getting some normalcy. Granted it will never be as it was before the cancer, but we have been given a fresh start to begin a whole new chapter in our lives.

EPILOGUE

Epilogue
The New Normal

Each day Terry wakes up just like billions of other people. The difference as each dawn comes is that she is one day closer to the first anniversary of her heart transplant.

Why is this anniversary so important, you ask? Because, even though she has received this precious gift, it does not come with a 100 percent, no-risk guarantee. Generally cardiac transplant patients suffer one to three episodes of rejection in the first year. Cases of acute rejection occur within the first three to six months and the incidence is significantly lower after this time. We have now passed that threshold. In fact, next week she will pass the nine-month mark. This does not mean she will not suffer some form of rejection. The fact is, according to the statistics, 50 to 80 percent experience at least one episode in their lifetime. In the first year, 18 percent of heart transplant deaths are the result of acute rejection and 22 percent are the result of the infections caused by the compromised immune system.[5] Hence, the reason for all the protocols I discussed earlier.

By year four and five, death rate by rejection is less than 10 percent. Terry will need to be monitored for rapidly progressing coronary heart disease in the arteries of the transplanted heart. This condition is known as allograft vasculopathy or CAV for short. CAV is a silent killer and occurs in 2 to 28 percent of patients in the first year after heart transplant and 40 to 70 percent of transplanted patients five years after transplant. Basically all the nerves to the heart are cut at the time of transplant, and it isn't possible to reconnect all those nerves when the new heart is in.

As you know when nerves are damaged or severed they do not heal or transmit signals from the brain. Sometimes the body will retrain other nerves to take over a particular function. With a transplant, you can't count on it. As a result, CAV progresses silently, sometimes rapidly. Affected patients don't feel the pain of angina and the symptoms associated with exertion, such as shortness of breath, excessive sweating, heartburn, nausea, light-headedness and fainting are often infrequent, atypical and can be misleading, Progressive heart failure, silent heart attack and sudden death are common.[6] There is also an increased possibility of certain cancers, primarily skin cancer, as a result of the prolonged use of the anti-rejection drugs.

As you can see, life it not as simple as it used to be. Even though Terry keeps getting stronger by the day, each day brings new challenges. If she has swelling, we add Lasik (the diuretic medication) to reduce the swelling. If her blood pressure is high, I call the hospital and ask that the transplant coordinator on call be paged. Within minutes the coordinator calls and gives us the appropriate instructions and we act accordingly. If her blood work shows her white blood cell count is low, I have to take her for a booster shot to jump start her bone marrow. Everything is still getting tweaked.

Sometimes Terry gets frustrated with all of this. Last Friday morning was one of these days. Her blood pressure monitor was not working properly and she got all upset. She started whining and complaining and this set me off. I always look at the glass as being half full while she looks at it as half empty. I called her an ingrate and started yelling. I told her, "You have been given this tremendous gift of life and you bitch over having to take your blood pressure twice a day? Do you hear yourself? I would bet your donor wouldn't mind taking her blood pressure if the roles were reversed!" This shut her up and got her thinking about how she was acting. I was so worked up I just grabbed my keys and went out for breakfast. Upon returning I was still fuming. This is unusual for me because I just let it out, calm down and move on. So I just went downstairs and spent the day working in my basement office. She knew I was really angry so she gave me my space. Saturday morning came and all returned to normal. She did her morning routine, we got dressed and went to the Farmers Market in Old Town Manassas. Yesterday was forgotten, the point was made.

* * *

Tomorrow is Wednesday and it's clinic day. This will be Terry's nine month checkup. The technician will draw blood to check for all the regular items plus some additional tests her primary doctor requested. Then she will have her monthly exam. If all is well, we will hear the now familiar response I am always happy to hear: "Your heart and lungs sure do sound boring." After we leave the clinic, we will go to the other lab so they can draw more blood to do the AlloMap®. This mapping will determine if she is experiencing any rejection. At both the clinic and at the lab she will have to wear a mask for protection. Hopefully late Friday afternoon we will receive a call from the clinic with good news. If this is the case, month nine will be behind us. If not, we will have more appointments next week.

* * *

Today's exam went as I just explained with one exception. Mary Beth Maydosz commented on Terry's tan. Terry replied, "Thank you. I've been sitting out on the deck."

That's when Mary Beth reminded her about no sun. The incidents of skin cancer are much higher in transplant patients. So she warned Terry to stay out of the sun and to use a good sunscreen and cover up if she had to be out.

Both places had trouble drawing blood from Terry today. Over the last five years her right arm has been poked so often her small veins are no longer in decent shape. They cannot use her left arm because of the lumpectomy.

Word of the book is working its way through the grapevine. Tonya told me she would like Julia Roberts to play her in the movie. Mary Beth gave me the name of an actress I never heard of.

I said, "Who?"

She gave the name again and it still rang no bells. Then she said, "You know, She's young, beautiful and blonde."

Upon hearing this I just remained silent.

Then she said, "You look and act just like my husband."

I replied, "One thing I learned as a husband is when in trouble, shut up. Do not dig yourself in deeper."

Both Terry and Mary Beth then shared a good laugh. As for the actress, I never heard of her. It's like *People Magazine*; every time I look at it, I know I'm getting older, because I don't recognize anyone in the magazine.

* * *

Here are portions of the update I emailed today to Terry's Heart list:

Today is May 4, 2012, our 44th wedding anniversary. We are celebrating, but not with a big party or anything like that. We just shared our day or at least most of it together. I attended a Prince William Chamber of Commerce breakfast and Terry had lunch with an old friend she hasn't seen in several years. Other than that, we spent the day with each other and in the evening we dined at our friend's restaurant. It was such a beautiful evening. We ate outside on the patio. At dinner I told Terry if she liked, to have a glass of wine and if she did I wouldn't let Mary Beth know (she's not supposed to have any form of alcohol for one year). After all, a 44th wedding anniversary is a milestone, especially in our case, with all we have been through these last five years. Plus we were celebrating the fact that Terry passed her nine-month post heart transplant anniversary. All of her test results from last week were great. Yesterday she received her reinstatement letter from the DMV that granted her unrestricted driving privileges. No more sending all the medical forms every four months for review.

I am still working on the book. I passed another milestone: 46,000 words (you have to love Microsoft Word for counting them for you). My plan is to finish with the one-year anniversary of her transplant.

REPONSES:

Happy Anniversary! I know you're happy for more than one reason. I'm glad to hear how well Terry is doing. Have a happy anniversary and a great weekend.
Terrific news, thank you for the update and happy anniversary!

Are you taking her out to Burger King for dinner like Mike M. takes his wife to celebrate their anniversary?
Fantastic! Back to a regular license, you're in real trouble now Joe!
Congratulations on your wedding anniversary and Terry's progress.

Happy Anniversary! Give Terry my best!!

Nice report Joe. I'm very happy for the both of you.

GREAT, GREAT NEWS! And Happy Anniversary all around!

Congratulations on the anniversary and God Bless both of you.
* * *

That is AWESOME news! We are looking forward to visiting with you and Terry in a couple of weeks. Make sure you have a cold beer or two waiting for me!

Happy Anniversary – 44 years, WOW!

It's almost midnight now. Terry went to bed about an hour or so ago. The house is quiet and little Eddie L. Barker is sleeping next to me on the couch. I'm just sitting here reflecting not only on today, but how fortunate we have been, especially these last three years. Had events gone in another direction the anniversary today would be quite different. Instead of being together I would have gone to the cemetery said a prayer and laid flowers on her grave. Say what you will, but she really has a Guardian Angel watching over her. These last five years, at just the right moment, the right person, the right professionals came into our lives. Individuals like her coworker, Phyllis, who pushed her to the nurse's office and was assertive with the nurse; all the friends and family for all their support and prayers, the many strangers in churches around the country who prayed for her. There was her primary doctor, who gave her the ultimatum that leads to the discovery of breast cancer at an early stage; the wonderful interventional radiologist at Inova Fair Oaks Hospital who safely removed the blood clot without her losing her leg. Then there is Dr. Thorn, the cardiologist at Prince William Hospital who literally saved her when she was basically two heart beats away from a pine box. All the wonderful people at Inova Heart and Vascular Institute at Inova Fairfax Hospital: the doctors, nurses and staff. Then we have the real unsung heroes of this, the organ donor and her family. Yes, this day could have been quite different. Thank you Lord for this day, and bless all these wonderful people.

* * *

Today is May 11, 2012, the Friday before Mother's Day and Terry went shopping by herself. She had 30 percent off coupons to Kohl's and they were burning a hole in her pocket. I really didn't care because she needed some new clothes. Terry really hasn't purchased anything for the last two years, plus it brightened her spirits. After all, what woman doesn't like to shop or get a bargain. Anyway, I carried the bags in when she got home. The shopping wore her out. So now both Terry and Eddie L. Barker are sound asleep on the loveseat. I received confirmation today of acceptance into an arts & crafts show in Myrtle Beach this summer. Now I can finalize the travel plans and we can combine work with a much needed mini-vacation. God willing, there will be no hospitalcations this summer!

* * *

Monday, May 21, and I am sitting here at the heart center while Terry has her ten-month heart biopsy and heart catheterization. The scheduling was moved up due to the Memorial Day holiday this weekend. As we were in the pre-op waiting for her to be wheeled in, her nurse, Grace, asked Terry, "How long have you both been married?" After hearing Terry's response, she commented, "You make such a cute couple." We started chuckling to each other. Yesterday while we were at brunch at a local restaurant, one of the wait staff told us the same thing. I told Terry I should see about getting a vanity plate for the car that would read CUTE-CPL.

Terry's now in the recovery area and we will have to wait for several hours before we can go home. She hates it when the procedure is scheduled for 11 a.m. or later. By the time they start it's usually after noon. Then by the time they finish and she is in recovery, she will not be able to eat until around 3 or 4 p.m. By then she is really starving after fasting since midnight. Mary Beth has come in and checked her out. She scolded Terry again about her tan and the importance of using sunscreen when she is outdoors. Failure to do so can result in a dermatologist removing a piece of nose here or a piece of the ear there. This week I will be sure to pick up a tube of sunscreen for her. I don't want half of the "CUTE-CPL" ruined.

* * *

Memorial Weekend has come and gone. My brother Augie and his family came down for the weekend. Terry had a wonderful time with my sister-in-law Eliz and my niece Jessica who recently turned 21. They went out shopping, went to see a chick flick and had lunch out. Over all it was a great four days. The only damper was that I was bitten by some insect which caused severe inflamed tendons in my left foot making me one big couch potato. Life has settled into what can be classified as mundane. After all that has transpired over the last five years it seems really weird not to be dealing with a major health issue.

* * *

Yesterday was the first Tuesday of the month. This means it's the support group monthly meeting at the heart center. The topic was post transplant care, and the different transplant nurse coordinators moderate the discussion. It was the first group meeting Terry has attended since before her transplant. At first she did not want to go but once there she enjoyed herself. Afterwards she told me she not only learned some new things but felt good that she was able to contribute to future transplantees. At the meeting we met a very nice young gentleman who is a personal trainer. I would guess he is in his mid-30s. He has had both left and right VADS since November 2011. He demonstrated a simple exercise program using a wall, chair or countertop to help VAD patients regain their strength and build core strength to help make carrying all the gear easier. In his case, its approximately 40 extra pounds. His attitude and outlook were unbelievable. Both Terry and I were both extremely impressed with this young man. Everyone we have met in this support group over the last two years has been very positive and motivated. This young man has taken it to a whole new level. He is still working full time plus being a dad and husband. This is no small accomplishment for someone with a VAD, but to do it with two VADs is unbelievable. We both said a prayer for him last night.

* * *

This morning at breakfast I had a conversation with JP, a friend of mine, and his son Matt. We were discussing death with dignity. During the conversation I mentioned on how Terry felt throughout her odyssey. I told him I didn't think I could go through what she endured. She never had any anxiety or fear. She had two open heart surgeries within a year. She always smiled and was upbeat and fearless before these surgeries. I shared with them the way she joked and what she told the medical staff as they rolled her into the operating room for her heart transplant.

JP told me, "It's because she a classy lady. You guys have something special. Remember the first time she came here for breakfast with you? She was completely comfortable and at ease. As one who met her for the first time, you could tell you both are completely at ease with each other, with total trust in each other. She knows you will let her do whatever she wants and will always have her back."

Later that afternoon I told Terry about my earlier conversation with JP. She responded by saying, "I never worried for two reasons. First, I knew that you were the one who always listened intently, took the notes, did the research, developed the questions, and interpreted the complex procedures for me. Second, I believe when I die, I know I will be going home. It will be peaceful, quiet and beautiful. I don't fear death. It's just a new beginning."

Even after 44 years of marriage, this woman continues to impress me.

* * *

It's almost 9 a.m. on June 14. We are arriving at Mullen Elementary School for our granddaughter Olivia's moving up ceremony from elementary to middle school. We arrived early to get a good seat. Wow, she is growing up so fast! As I sat there, I remembered her first day of school. She was so full of piss and vinegar with her head high and a big confident smile on her face, toting a backpack that looked bigger than she was. On her sixth birthday, I brought in a birthday cake and juice drinks for her Kindergarten class. I remembered all the different field trips I chaperoned over the years; the times I picked her up from the nurse's office because she was sick or the times I delivered her lunch because she forgot it or the times I just joined her for lunch in the cafeteria. Most importantly I watched as Terry viewed and enjoyed the entire program. At each of life's small milestones we shared these past 11 months I rejoice in the fact we are sharing them together. At the same time I can't help but to think of the darker side had we not been so blessed. These simple events shared together mean so much more to us now. The Lord has been good to us and he continues to spread his grace upon us.

* * *

Today is Father's Day and Terry and I are spending it quietly. She took me out for brunch this morning and I cut the grass after we got home. It's now mid-afternoon and Terry's taking a nap on the loveseat. Eddie L. Barker is sleeping on her stomach.

I decided it was time to do my usual Father's Day ritual. I take Tim Russert's two books off the self and reread various chapters. In his first book, *Big Russ and I,* there are so many shared memories since he and I grew up in Buffalo at the same time: Tim in south Buffalo; me on Buffalo's west side. The similarities in his stories and the lessons learned from his dad have so many parallels with those I learned from my dad. His second book, *Wisdom of our Fathers,* brings me to tears because he used my dad's picture and two of his sayings in the book. Dad's picture is featured on page 179, starting the chapter titled *"Memories."* As I look at Dad's picture and begin to read the chapter, I think of Dad and how I wish I could have just one more day with him. I am a prime example of what Mark Twain once said: "When I was a boy of 14, my father was so ignorant I could hardly stand to have the old man around. But when I got to be 21, I was astonished how much the old man had learned in seven years."

Dad had a saying for virtually every occasion. His favorite was, "Hugs are free. One day when I'm not around, you're going to want one." Boy, there have been at least a thousand plus times these past five years when I could have really used one of his hugs. Instead, in each of these difficult situations, I would ask myself, "How would Dad handle it?" Then I would form my path using that as a basis.

* * *

It's time again for Terry's monthly clinic visit. We are now at Month 11. Mary Beth was very impressed with how she is doing. They drew blood as usual, and had a difficult time finding a vein. After the clinic appointment we went to the lab so more blood could be drawn for the AlloMap®. When she came out she had bandages everywhere. She told me they finally had to take the blood from her left hand. That upset me because they are not to do anything on her left side because of her lumpectomy. Now we wait for the results. Mary Beth's first call gave us the results from the hospital blood work. Terry's Prograf level is high. Mary Beth instructed me to lower her dose from 3mg to 1.5mg daily. Next week she will need more blood drawn to make sure everything's okay. The AlloMap® results take longer; hopefully we will have the results by the end of the week. Mary Beth's second call will let us know if there are signs of rejection based on the AlloMap®. Next month, on the one year anniversary, they already have her scheduled for a left and right heart catheterization. This will be an all day event at the hospital. We need to be there at 9 a.m. and with any luck; we will leave around 6 p.m., just in time for rush hour and a long drive home in slow-moving traffic.

* * *

On Friday I received an email from Mary Beth with the AlloMap® results. The test revealed that Terry's score translated to a 99.3 percent prognosis of not experiencing any rejection. The rest of the month was quiet – well, almost quiet. Our daughter Kelly interviewed for a job in Charlotte, North Carolina. Kelly has had several interviews in North Carolina over the last year and we didn't think much about it. This time it seemed different, so Terry and I talked about what we would do if Kelly got the job and moved with Olivia.

Terry was surprised by my answer. I quickly responded by saying, "We just pack up and move to Rockhill, South Carolina." Rockhill is just over the state line from Charlotte.

Terry said, "Have you talked to Kelly?"

"No, why?" I asked.

"Kelly suggested the exact same thing to me," Terry said. "Joe, you would really move?"

"Yes," I said. "We have nothing holding us here in Virginia."

* * *

Today is July 3, 2012 and we are on our first three-day getaway in years. Currently we are in Spencer, North Carolina for Norfolk Southern Corporation's 30th Anniversary two-day celebration, featuring a display of all 20 locomotives in their heritage fleet. For a railfan, this is like dying and going to Heaven. NS painted 20 diesel engines fresh from the engine shops in the original color scheme of all the railroads which were merged into Norfolk Southern. To see them all in one place at the

193

same time is a once-in-a-lifetime opportunity as they all will return to service as freight engines. While I photographed to my heart's content, Terry sat in the shade or in one of the air-conditioned buildings as it was extremely hot. She met several other railfan widows like Linda from Pittsburgh, Pennsylvania and Kathy from Fairfax, Virginia. We both had a wonderful day. We were together and enjoying our first getaway. Kelly called her mom and told her she got the job and would be moving to Charlotte. She would start the job July 23. This meant she had a lot to do in the next two-and-a-half weeks.

On the way out Tuesday evening, Terry turned her ankle. I'm hoping it's only sprained, but she refuses to go have it checked out. As we awoke on July 4th, Terry's ankle is no better and she continues to refuse medical attention. She decided to stay in the room and rest it. After I got her all squared away, I left for festivities. Upon returning later in the afternoon, I found her right where I left her in bed. Terry struggled to get dressed so we could go to dinner. When we then attempted to make our way down the hall, she only made it six feet before we had to stop. The pain was too bad. I wanted to call 911 because I knew she had more than just a sprain, and I worried about getting her off the second floor of the motel and into the car the next morning. She made it very clear she wanted no part of 911. I left her in the room and went to get carryout for her. On the way, I stopped at a drug store and bought an ACE bandage to wrap her foot. Upon returning I made an ice pack for her to ice the foot while she ate. Thirty seconds later she was whining it was too cold for her and I took it off. Here's a woman who underwent two open heart surgeries – one, a heart transplant, and she could not handle a little ice.

  * * *

Morning has come. It's time to pack up and head for home. Terry's foot is no better. Of course if you ask, she claims it's fine, everything's okay. She didn't walk around the bed. She slid her butt across the bed to get dressed without standing up. Getting Terry down the hall, the flight of stairs, and into the SUV was no small chore. We looked like the Three Stooges minus one. If someone had videoed this, and posted it to the Internet, it would have gone viral. I told her we were going to the local hospital's emergency room. She fought me, tooth and nail, refusing to go. She just wanted to come home. We compromised. We would go home and upon getting there, she was going to the doctor's.

On the way home I called my podiatrist's office and got an appointment for the late afternoon. Once at the doctor's office, they took a series of x-rays. What they discovered was a cracked fibula and the metatarsal bone of the second toe is broke just below the tarsometatarsal joint. Dr. Bennett set her toe, taped her foot and put her in a walking cast.

I said to Terry: "I don't want to say I told so, but I TOLD YOU SO!"

I guess our uneventful summer is now out the window. This was to be the summer of no hospitals and no doctors. As they say, it looked good on paper; so much for the plans on the drawing board. Now she does not want to go to Myrtle Beach with a cast on her foot.

Oh, well, that's tomorrow's battle.

On the way home we stopped at Kelly's to pick Eddie. Kelly had already planned her move. A friend could get her all the boxes she would need except wardrobe boxes. She reserved a truck from U-Haul and also labor to load here and unload there. Nikki and Sean drove down from Erie on Monday, July 16 and stayed at our house. Tuesday the truck was loaded and Sean drove the truck to Charlotte where they were met the crew to unload. Needless to say it made for a very long day. Sean and Nikki drove home on Wednesday.

* * *

Today is Monday, July 23. We had to be at the heart center at 8:30 a.m. for several reasons. First, the results from Terry's blood tests last week revealed her Prograf level was low, so the transplant coordinator upped her dosage level. Terry needed to have blood drawn to check if her Prograf level is back to where it needs to be. Second, as we approach the one year anniversary of her transplant, Terry is scheduled to have a right and left heart catheterization plus the heart biopsy. Think of it as buying a new car and this is your 12,000-mile check up to make sure everything is operating at peak performance. It is all part of her one year evaluation.

The procedure was scheduled for 11 a.m., but just before they were to roll her into the catheterization lab she was bumped due to an emergency. So now we are in a holding pattern until a catheterization lab becomes available. After the procedure she will need four hours of bed rest before the staff allows her to get up. If everything went on schedule we would leave here around 4:30 to 5 p.m. Now that we are in the holding pattern, the Lord only knows when we will leave here. Needless to say it makes for a long day. All of this reminds me of the time I spent in the Air Force where you hurry up and wait. Terry is sound asleep right now because of the medication they gave her for the procedure, so instead of sitting in this hard straight back chair any longer I'm moving to the lounge area to have a cup of coffee and sit on one of the nicer lounge chairs. I know my back will be grateful.

While waiting, I went to speak with Deanna, the transplant financial coordinator. We have been billed by the hospital for some transplant-related procedures for which we should not have to pay. The way our insurance is set up, anything having to do with the transplant is covered 100 percent for the first year. Someone in the billing department submitted the bill under the wrong medical code and the insurance company is treating it as a medical claim rather than as a transplant claim. I have been trying to get this resolved since April. Hopefully we can make some progress this time around.

It's now 2:35 p.m. and I'm sitting in the recovery room with Terry. She is sound asleep. The procedure went off without any problems. Hopefully by Friday all the results will be in. I have to mention, the chairs in the recovery rooms are a step up from the pre-op chairs. These have a padded seat. My backside greatly appreciates this small comfort. It's now a few minutes past 3 p.m. and Terry woke up for about 30 seconds, spoke a few words to the nurse and was off to sleepy land again. As I'm sitting here I can't help but think how things were a year ago. Sometimes it feels like any eternity. Other times it feels like just yesterday. Terry has come so far in this past year. Granted, it will never be the way it was before this all started five years ago and I wonder if it's really not better now. Now we appreciate each other and each day more deeply. We don't take life or each other for granted. We learned how precious life really is and to enjoy each day. Each day is a blessing. Yesterday is in the past and we can't change anything. Tomorrow is the future with no guarantees we will see it. We only have today to love, to enjoy, and to live.

* * *

Today is Thursday, July 26, 2012, almost to the minute that we received the call that a heart may be available. I can remember as if it just happened, like a moment cemented in your mind forever. It's like remembering where and what you were doing when President John F. Kennedy was shot or when the highjacked planes hit the World Trade Center's twin towers, the Pentagon and Flight 93 went down in Pennsylvania.

A whole year has passed with its ups and downs. I have watched Terry evolve from knocking on death's door to a healthy vibrant woman with a whole lot of living yet to do. We received a call from the clinic. Terry's left and right heart catheterization numbers were great, the biopsy was another 1, with no signs of rejection. The only downer was her Prograf level for some reason keeps dropping. So I have to increase her daily dosage by another .05mg. Next week she will have to have blood drawn to check her Prograf level. All the tests she took this week are leading up to what is the Anniversary Checkup. She still needs to have an electrocardiogram and an echocardiogram done. Both tests are scheduled for August 7. Also on that date, Terry has been asked to be part of the transplant panel at the August meeting of the support group. This was the same form of meeting our daughters attended last August. Now it's our turn to give back and relieve some other family's fears and anxiety, and to demonstrate there really is a light at the end of the tunnel.

On Sunday we leave for a working vacation at Myrtle Beach (I work while Terry vacations). We will stop over to visit our daughter and granddaughter in Charlotte. I will be doing an arts & crafts show while Terry visits with her friend, Phyllis.

* * *

Heart Update First Anniversary

Exactly one year ago at this time Terry hopped on the gurney and we were off to the operating room pre-op, which began this past year's rollercoaster ride. Like all rollercoaster rides this one had its ups and downs as you all know. Sometimes we just clicked, clicked, clicked our way very slowly; other times we were 60 mph. In the end, it has been a terrific ride. *Terry is doing GREAT!* This past week she had a left and right heart catheterization and all her blood tests were completed. The new heart is working wonderfully with no rejection. On August 7 she is scheduled for an electrocardiogram and an echocardiogram as part of her one-year check up. On a lower note, Terry broke her foot on July 3. Yesterday we found out she will need surgery to repair it. The metatarsal bone of the second toe shifted after it was set three weeks ago and during the surgery, Dr. Bennett will reset it and install a pin in it. We just can't escape hospitals and doctors in the summer.

This will be the last official heart update I will be sending out. For a complete recap of our whole journey, including details that weren't in the heart updates, you will just have to read the book, which is written from all my notes, journals and email updates, and wraps up with the first year anniversary.

Terry and I wish to thank each and every one of you for all your prayers, support and well wishes throughout this entire odyssey. Without you guys, I don't think we would be where we are today.

Responses:

All great news.

Joe, not only is she doing great, she looks GREAT! I look forward to a copy of the book signed by the Squirt!

Great news about Terry's Heart status. I hope the EKG & Echo go as well. Sorry to hear about the broken foot and hope the surgery is successful. My son Scott just had a pin put in his broken hand after suffering a bad ATV collision with a tree.

God bless! So happy to hear that Terry is doing amazing. Tell her hello from me

YEAH Terry! Great way to start off the day with such, well except for the foot, news! Will continue to keep you in my prayers cause it doesn't hurt. Good luck with the foot op!

Happy anniversary to Terry and to both of you! Congratulations on reaching your personal goal of finishing your book today! I believe reading about your journey will help many others face their own journeys and know that they aren't alone, that they too have guardian angels and a support network of family and friends to help them through, if they just reach out for them. It's been great reading all your updates and seeing how God has been working through you. Cherish each day!

Great news. Give Terry a big hug for me

You guys have surely had a rollercoaster ride this past year. I am so delighted that it has ended on a high note (except the broken foot part). Keep up the good work, Terry!

What a great report Joe. Sorry about the foot Terry. Stay well!! Blessings.

Praise God for His faithfulness and for Terry's new heart and health. Thanks for allowing us to be part of this journey with you both.

Throughout the entire process of writing this book, I thought about just how I would end it. Would I end it by reporting on a really high note and big celebration? As the actual day arrived, July 27, 2012, all I can think of is the fact that Terry and I have had 365 more days together. The celebration was a private family time together. Our daughters both sent their mom a first year birthday card celebrating their mother's one year anniversary. Terry and I shared a glass of wine tonight to mark this amazing year. Eddie L. Barker, who added so much unconditional love in our healing journey, was there to share the event nestled in Terry's lap.

Our lives will never be like they were before all this started five years ago, but I do believe they are far better. We have learned to appreciate each day and do our best to live each day to the fullest. I really get emotional thinking about what could have been, had Terry not fallen, which in turn sent the blood clot south to her leg and not up her aorta. What if we never met Dr. Thorn and all the absolutely wonderful doctors, nurses, medical technicians and staff of Inova Heart and Vascular Institute? What if we had not experienced all the strangers who prayed for her across the country, and the friends and family whose support kept my morale up even at the darkest moments?

I'm just grateful to have one more day together with my wife. I guess that in itself is the greatest celebration of all. It's the celebration of life. I am eternally grateful to the organ donor and her family whose sacrifice made this all possible. Every morning as I awake I ask the good Lord to grant a special place in his kingdom for Terry's donor; and to bring peace and consolation to her family. Each day we wake up and have one more day to be together, to share, to love, and be thankful for all our blessings we have. For her Guardian Angel who watched over her and the Good Lord who made all this possible, thank you.

BEGINNING
Post Script:
I retired in October 2012 closed my business, we sold our house in Manassas and in fact moved to Rock Hill, South Carolina on December 13, 2012. Terry continues to do great all of her two year anniversary test results were Fantastic. We have become very involved with Saint Anne's Catholic Church here in Rock Hill. For us it's away to say thank you Jesus and to give back to the community.

INDEX

Index

This is the summary of a paper published and copyrighted in 1977 by the American Association of Cancer Research. The authors are F.P.Mettler, D.M. Young and J.M. Ward.

Adriamycin-induced Cardiotoxicity (Cardiomyopathy and Congestive Heart Failure) in Rats

By _F. P. Mettler, D. M. Young, and J. M. Ward_

Comparative Pathology Section, Laboratory of Toxicology, Experimental Therapeutics Program, Division of Cancer Treatment, National Cancer Institute, NIH, Bethesda, Maryland 20014

Summary

The recent development of numerous analogs of the anthracycline class of oncolytic agents has resulted in an urgent need for a standardized, accurate, reproducible, and cost-effective system for cardiotoxicity testing. The present studies were designed to determine the feasibility of using the rat as a model for induction of the chronic type of cardiotoxicity (_i.e._, cardiomyopathy and congestive heart failure). Adriamycin (ADR) was administered to rats at doses of 1 to 2 mg/kg/week for 10 to 14 weeks. The majority of ADR-treated rats developed cardiomyopathy from 3 to 23 weeks after the last injection. Forty to 70% of those rats with cardiomyopathy had gross evidence of congestive heart failure (pleural effusions, ascites, hepatomegaly, cardiomegaly). Histological myocardial changes consisted of myocyte vacuolation and degeneration, interstitial edema, and mild fibroplasia. In addition, damage to atrial ganglion cells was evident in several rats. Ultrastructural alterations involved sarcoplasmic disruption with distentions of subcellular organelles and loss of myofilaments. Extracardiac toxic effects of ADR (nephrotoxicity, myelosuppression, enteropathy, arrested osteogenesis) were minor and were observed more frequently at higher cumulative doses.

The results of the present study suggest that the rat model is an accurate, reproducible, and cost-effective system for large-scale cardiotoxicity testing of analogs of ADR and daunorubicin.

©1977 American Association for Cancer Research.

For more information, go to: http://cancerres.aacrjournals.org/content/37/8_Part_1/2705.abstract

---

[1] *Slogan is used with the permission of the Timex Corporation.

[2] ©1977 American Association for Cancer Research, F.P.Mettler, D.M. Young and J.M. Ward, authors. [see Index]

[3] Prayer written by Carol D. July 28, 2011

[4] [3] The Prayer of Humble Access is a prayer immediately prior to communion in Mass.

[5] Statistics provided by Wolters Kluwer Health, www.uptodate.com

[6] Paraphrased from Wolters Kluwer Health,

Amazing

www.uptodate.com